Office YOGA

Julie Friedeberger has practised yoga for twenty years. She holds the British Wheel of Yoga Teachers' Diploma and the teaching certificates of the Dharma Yoga Centre and the Bodyworkshop. In this book she shares her experience of yoga and of working life, and her knowledge of applying the one to the other.

Julie Friedeberger is currently at work, in collaboration with her teacher, Swami Dharmānanda Saraswati, on a handbook entitled *A Manual of Basic Yoga Practices*. She lives in London with her husband, the painter Klaus Friedeberger.

Office
YOGA

Tackling tension with simple stretches you can do at your desk

Julie Friedeberger

Thorsons
An Imprint of HarperCollins*Publishers*

Thorsons
An Imprint of GraftonBooks
A Division of HarperCollins*Publishers*
77-85 Fulham Palace Road
Hammersmith, London W6 8JB

Published by Thorsons 1991

10 9 8 7 6 5 4 3 2 1
© 1991 Julie Friedeberger

Julie Friedeberger asserts the moral right to
be identified as the author of this work

A CIP catalogue record for this book
is available from the British Library

ISBN 0 7225 2537 0

Printed in Great Britain by
HarperCollinsManufacturing, Glasgow

For my husband, Klaus
and my teacher, Swami Dharmānanda Saraswati

*Whoever has helped us to a larger understanding is entitled to
our gratitude for all time.*

Norman Douglas

ACKNOWLEDGEMENTS

Many friends have helped me along the path of yoga to the place where I can share something of what I know in this book. I am grateful to all of them; but I especially want to acknowledge and thank those who have taught me: Iris Reece, Stella Cherfas and Jack London, Tony Hurley, Barbara Dale (whose generous help has made it a better book), Brian Hately, Angela Thompson, Ken Thompson, John Cain, and Swami Dharmānanda Saraswati.

I am grateful to my students for giving me the opportunity and the privilege of teaching; and for showing me that this book was needed. Among them, special thanks are due to Hedda Beeby who, with her colleagues at Shared Experience, welcomed our classes to their wonderful studio space; to Clare Ford, for believing in the book and for editing it; and to Nick Bartlett and Billy Crowson, for so beautifully and accurately demonstrating the movements for the illustrations.

Lucy Su's lovely drawings have enhanced the book's appeal and its usefulness, and I am grateful to her for her contribution.

Most of all, my thanks and love to Klaus and Swamiji, to whom the book is dedicated.

Contents

Preface

This book is based on yoga, a system of physical, mental and spiritual development which originated in India at least 3,000 years ago. Its roots lie in Hindu philosophy, and its aim is to bring about balance and harmony on every level of one's being, by means of techniques which have been tested and proved over thousands of years, not only in India but by practitioners all over the world.

In this book, some of the basic practices and underlying principles of yoga are applied to working life. It is a kind of survival handbook for the desk-bound: a practical manual of simple yoga-based movements which can be done at the desk, a few minutes at a time throughout the day, to help relieve the tension and stress of working life.

But although it is an essentially practical book, I think – I hope – that it is true to the spirit of yoga.

Office Yoga is meant for anyone whose working hours are spent mainly at a desk, whether in an office or at home. Students, writers, draughtspeople and designers – anyone whose work requires a great deal of sitting – will find it helpful too. It can also be used by anyone who, for whatever reason, is unable to exercise from a standing position.

You will be able to use this book whether or not you have practised yoga before. If you are new to yoga, I hope you will find it clear, comprehensible and useful. Possibly it will inspire you to go further – for yoga is there to help us to fulfill our potential as human beings, and the possibilities are vast.

If you have had some yoga experience – if you have attended classes, and/or practised on your own, or are quite adept – you are probably already aware of the importance and value of bringing yoga as much as possible into your daily life. I hope you will find in this book some new ways and means of doing this.

Introduction

If you work in an office, you probably experience physical tension from time to time (if not most of the time). It's also quite likely that you experience mental tension: the result of your continual effort to deal with the pressures of work and with the demands that are made upon you.

You have my sympathies. In my own thirty-odd years of doing various jobs behind various desks I have experienced my fair share of office tension, and I am fully aware of how draining and debilitating it can be. I know the insidious effect it can have on the quality of your life – not only at work, but on the rest of it, the part outside work. And I also know that it is possible to tackle it: to relieve it when it takes hold, and even to prevent it taking hold at all.

The ache between the shoulder blades, the pain in the neck, the stiff lower back, the sore eyes, the feeling of shattered exhaustion at the end of a long, fraught day – which a student of mine has described as 'concussed' – may be your familiar, unwelcome companions, as they have been mine. They may have come to seem inevitable to you: occupational hazards, part of the job.

But they aren't inevitable. There is a great deal you can do about them, as I have learned, and as I hope to show you in this book.

No-one is exempt. Whatever your job – computer programmer, receptionist, secretary, designer, manager, or company chairman – you are vulnerable to the conditions I've described, and have probably experienced them. Office life *is* stressful and tension-inducing.

There are several reasons for this.

Office life is sedentary
The human body is made for movement and activity, and suffers when deprived of it. Joints maintain their mobility, and muscles their elasticity, only if they are used. And all the body systems – respiratory, circulatory, digestive, etc – need movement if they are to function efficiently. Movement is natural and necessary, but most office jobs seem to require you to sit for long periods in a more or less fixed position.

You sit at a desk which may not be the right height for you and which, unless it has a sloping surface, is not at the proper angle for comfortable working. You sit in a chair which, unless you are very lucky, has not been designed for correct, comfortable sitting. All this adds up to a sure recipe for neck-ache, back-ache, head-ache, eye-ache and brain-ache.

Office life deprives you of vital oxygen

You need fresh air and a plentiful supply of oxygen as well as exercise, but because you are indoors most of the time you scarcely ever get any – especially if your working environment is air-conditioned. This, combined with the fact that you possibly do not breathe fully and deeply (few people do) means that you do not get a sufficient oxygen supply, and also that you don't fully expel toxins from your system. This affects your physical health, your mental and emotional balance, your concentration and your temper.

Office life is emotionally wearing

You are closely confined for upwards of eight hours a day with other people who are also trying to cope with these conditions. Some may be better off than others. The chairman may have a better chair than the receptionist, and a private office with a window that can be opened. The secretary may have more opportunities to move around the building and get more exercise than the manager. Essentially, though, you are all in the same boat: sitting uncomfortably and for too long at a stretch; more or less deprived of vital oxygen, and consequently often tense and irritable.

You all have to cope with one another as well as with your work and your working conditions, so at times your working environment may feel more like a madhouse or a zoo than a community of rational human beings. In times of stress you may get on one another's nerves, bite one another's heads off, snap at and score off one another. Possibly you contribute to the atmosphere yourself – not only by behaving like this, but also by regarding others as responsible for creating the situation and yourself as a victim of it, and by putting the blame on others for how you feel at the end of the day.

Office life can generate anxiety

If for any reason you feel insecure in your job – perhaps because you work in a highly competitive industry, or for an institution vulnerable to government cuts, or because you don't get on with your boss – the resulting anxiety creates further difficulties for you.

If your company is the scene of 'office politics' and power struggles (from which everyone suffers whether personally involved or not) you may well feel as bruised and battered at the end of the day as though you had spent it in the thick of battle.

You have to get to the office and back
If you work in a big town and live on its outskirts, your working day is sandwiched between struggles with rush-hour traffic or the crowds on public transport, and with inevitable delays in the form of traffic holdups and train cancellations. On a bad day, you may arrive at work infuriated and steaming, or in an exhausted heap, feeling that you've already had your fill of hassle. And you may reach home in the evening too tired to do anything but eat your dinner and fall into bed.

All these conditions are difficult enough to cope with even if you find your work fulfilling; even if you are doing what you want to be doing and are satisfied with the way your career is progressing. If you don't like your work – if you are bored or feel under-valued; if you are frustrated in your ambition or 'stuck' in a job you feel you can't leave; or if you have been over-promoted into a job that is beyond your present abilities – you have additional problems.

Of course, no-one experiences all of these trying conditions all of the time. But we all experience some of them some of the time, and because they are all *extra* to the work we are doing and the problems we are paid to solve, we don't even think about them very much. We just put up with them, grit our teeth and battle on, paying the price in all sorts of ways as tension and stress accumulate.

My own work, in publishing, has always required me to sit a great deal, doing jobs involving close, detailed work such as proof-reading. The physical aspect of 'office tension' is all too familiar to me: I know what it is to feel sore and knotted at the end of a busy day.

I actually like working in an office. I like the excitements of publishing, and I especially like the companionship and cameraderie of like-minded people which I've been lucky enough to have. For the past six years I have worked in an environment which is probably almost unique: a medium-sized firm in which people value and support one another and in which there is no back-stabbing (or even biting) – a real fellowship of responsible adults working together in reasonable harmony most of the time. Yet even here, I have experienced my share of stress: deadlines to be met, conflicting priorities, sheer pressure of work most of the time, and so on. All this, as well as the physical tension, has had to be coped with.

What has helped me to cope is that I have practised yoga for twenty years. During that time I have tried to apply my knowledge of yoga – not only of the movements and postures, but also of yoga's underlying principles - to my life as a whole. Yoga has changed my life for the better in every way, and has in fact become its guiding force. In my working life it has been a special kind of help, in easing tension and dealing with stress.

When I began to teach yoga, at a centre in central London, I found that the students who came to my first lunchtime and early morning classes were in situations similar to mine. They worked in offices, and they all – secretaries, administrators, department heads, directors – felt that they were under pressure and wanted to do something about it. This was, for most, the main motivation for coming to yoga: they wanted to learn to relax, and to cope better with the tension and stress they were experiencing. I knew that yoga could help them, but it seemed to me that I ought to be able to bring my own working experience to bear in my teaching, to give them specific help with the tensions and stresses that seem to arise so particularly out of working in an office.

I devised a series of workshops in which I introduced the students to simple, yoga-based movements, coordinated with breathing, that can be performed from a sitting position, without leaving one's desk. I called them 'Office Yoga', and they were useful: the students enjoyed them, and reported that they were able to use what they had learned at work.

An accompanying handout, reminding them of the exercises and how to practise them, was the germ of this book. I began to think that such a book was needed, and would be welcomed, and would be helpful. So I have written it. In it, I would like to share what I know about handling the stress of office life; and to pass on what my practice of yoga has taught me, in the hope that the practical advice and the insights I am able to offer will help you, too, to cope more effectively with the pressures you are under; so that the eight or more hours you spend at work each day can be happier, better hours; so that your working life can be more comfortable, more enjoyable and less wearing; and so that you feel the benefit in your *whole* life.

You will be able to help yourself more than you might think possible. For example, there are simple changes you can make on a purely practical level to improve the quality of your working life.

The first chapter tells you how to assess your working environment and your equipment – your chair, your desk, your lighting etc – and how to improve it. Some of the simplest adjustments, like changing the position of a lamp or the height of a chair, can make an appreciable difference to your comfort and well-being. This chapter also explains how to sit. Even if you think you know how to sit, please don't skip this part: it is important. Sitting well will make the biggest overall difference to your well-being, because how you sit affects not only the relationship of all the parts of your body, but, even more importantly, your breathing.

The correct sitting position is the starting point for all the exercises in Chapters 2, 3 and 4. These exercises can all be done sitting in your chair, at your desk, to relieve tension, aches and pains; replenish your vitality; and make you feel generally better throughout the day.

If you feel hesitant about calling attention to yourself at first, you will find that you can do quite a few of the exercises in these chapters unobtrusively, without anyone else being aware that you are doing them. Start with these, and move on to the others as you gain confidence. If it causes a little hilarity, there's nothing wrong with that, and you will probably find your colleagues joining you before long! You might like to try the exercises at home first, so that you'll know which ones you will feel happy about starting with at work, and so you'll know how to do them.

Chapter 5 is about breathing. Awareness of breath, and the coordination of movement and breath, are the essence of yoga. This chapter explains this principle; and also explains why it is so important to breathe well, and how yoga can help. This leads on to Chapter 6, and some movement and breathing sequences which are performed from a standing position. If you are able to find a quiet corner to disappear to for a few minutes, or perhaps a quiet time when there aren't many people around, you will find these especially helpful for stretching your whole body, stimulating your breathing, restoring your energy, and generally banishing the cobwebs.

These six chapters are the 'practical' part of the book. The exercises will help you to alleviate muscular tension when it hits you, or, better still, to head it off before it hits you. All the exercises are coordinated with breathing – for which instruction is given – and this will benefit your circulation and improve your concentration. You may also find that practising them helps you to maintain higher energy levels, and that you approach your work more enthusiastically.

The seventh chapter is about the 'tops and tails' of your working day. It suggests some possibilities for making better use of the time you spend travelling to and from work, and of your lunch time.

Chapter 8 summarizes what you can do throughout your day to relieve the tension you may experience in specific situations, and what to do when you are too busy and fraught to think what to do!

If this book is your introduction to yoga, and you want to take it further, the final chapter offers suggestions for finding a yoga class and advice on practising yoga at home. If your interest in yoga deepens, you may want to do more reading about it. There is a reading list at the end of the book.

You will soon become aware that yoga offers a great deal more than physical exercise. That particular aspect is the one most of us in the West are acquainted with, and the movements and postures of yoga do indeed provide excellent exercise. They work systematically on the muscles and joints to develop not just suppleness, but also strength, stamina, balance, and resistance to injury. They encourage the proper functioning of all the body systems, and assist in the elimination of toxins. But they also develop mental and emotional, as well as physical, steadiness and balance: in yoga, you train your mind as well as your body.

Yoga is really an all-embracing system for the creation of balance and harmony on all levels of one's being: physical, emotional, mental and spiritual. Yoga practice is a journey of self-discovery. The goal of that journey is the full realization of one's potential. If you start on that journey you will develop and change. Yoga practice can help you to become healthier, more relaxed and more content; stronger and more self-disciplined. It can give you greater vitality and optimism, and help you to approach the problems of life in a more positive, more creative way.

Alongside the difficulties and frustrations which occasionally arise out of our relations with other people at work, the physical pains in the neck can seem trivial. But you will find it easier to deal with these, too, as you grow more stable and more aware, and as your outlook changes.

What we are, how we develop as individuals, and what we become, is very largely determined by our own attitude, our own thoughts. We have a certain degree of control over our situation and our circumstances, (although this may be more, or less, than we think). We have no control over other people, nor should we want it. But, potentially, we do have complete control over our own attitude and our own thoughts; over how we respond to situations and to people. This is as true in our working lives as it is in our personal relationships. We can change: and once we understand this, the possibilities for improving the quality of our lives and the lives of those around us are vast.

Yoga shows us the way to this transformation, and gives us the means of bringing it about.

Chapter 1
Sitting

Whatever your job, your responsibilities, or your position in your company, it's a fair assumption that the thing you do most of is sitting.

Poor posture, whether standing or sitting, is both tiring and unhealthy, because it demands unnecessary work of your muscles, strains your bones and ligaments, restricts your breathing, impedes your circulation and interferes with your digestion. It is vital, therefore, that you sit well. First you need to take a critical look at your equipment: your chair, your work surface and your lighting. Then you need to look at yourself and at how you sit.

Your chair
Very few chairs are designed for good sitting. Decent, well-designed office chairs do exist, but they are very expensive, and it's unlikely that you have one. However, you will almost certainly be able to improve the one you've been issued with.

If you have been given a chair that is broken, wobbly, or even mildly derelict, ask for it to be repaired or replaced with one that is in good condition. Don't put up with a chair that cannot be adjusted to the right height for you, or that is so skew-whiff that your spine is always being pulled out of line with the effort of sitting in it. Your health will suffer and so will your work.

Conventional office chairs are usually height-adjustable. Make quite sure that the height of your chair is right for your body, and also right in relation to the height of your table or desk. This should be such that your body does not have to make adjustments that are harmful to its structure. You need to be able to position yourself over your work without having to collapse your spine or your chest, round your back, hunch your shoulders, or contract your neck.

Finding the best position may take you several days, as you experiment with various heights, but do persevere until it feels right. Even a small difference in height adjustment can make a big difference to your comfort. If you are short, you will probably find, as I do, that you need to sit fairly high – but then your feet will dangle, which will unbalance you and strain your back. Your feet need to be firm and flat on the ground, so put something under them: a couple of telephone directories, or a stool, or an empty letter tray.

If you are tall, adjustment will depend on whether your length is mostly in your upper body (in which case you should experiment with the height of your seat to bring yourself into the right relationship to your work) or in your legs (in which case you may need to place your feet further away from you, with a wider angle between your calves and your thighs).

Long-legged people often wind their legs around the legs of chairs, possibly for someplace to put them. Do try to avoid doing this: it will cut off your circulation. Whatever your height, avoid crossing your legs for the same reason.

Although an armchair is widely regarded as a status symbol, an acknowledgement that its occupier has moved up in the world, a chair without arms is really better for you. Using the arms of a chair to 'rest' your elbows and forearms almost invariably encourages you to lift your shoulders, especially if you are short in the upper body. The muscles of your neck, shoulders and upper back then work needlessly, creating tension. As most physical tension begins in this area anyway, the last thing you need is to manufacture more. You should try to keep your shoulders back and down at all times, and rest your hands in your lap when you aren't using them.

The Scandinavian kneeling chairs have become popular over the last ten years or so, mainly through their cheaper imitations available through mail order houses. I have mixed feelings about them. They allow you to sit with your hips higher than your knees, which encourages an upright spine. If you slump, you are more likely to realize it and correct yourself. This gives your internal organs more room so that they function better, and keeps your chest open and your ribcage free so that you breathe better. However, your legs are kept in a fixed position, which may lead to stiff knee joints; and there is considerable pressure on the shins, which is uncomfortable if you sit for a long time at a stretch.

If you are going to use a kneeling chair, make a point of getting up and moving around as often as you can. And get one that is height adjustable and has casters, so you can change position easily: most models are not suitable for office use, and the few that are are the (expensive) Scandinavian versions.

Much better, although even more expensive, are the Labomatic* chairs, made by Labofa. The back rest gives correct support for the lower back, and the seat height automatically positions the seat to suit your lower leg length. The seat itself is slightly tilted, which raises your hips higher than your knees, reducing pressure on your spine and allowing it to extend.

Your work surface

The height of your work surface should be such as to enable you to hold your shoulders back and down. You will have to achieve this mainly by adjusting the height of your chair, as there is not a great deal you can do about the height of your desk. Once you have got this right, you should consider the angle of your work in relation to your eyes.

The use of a horizontal surface for writing and reading encourages you to slouch forward, as your eyes try to find a comfortable distance and angle relationship with your work. A sloping surface brings the work into the right relationship with your vision, enabling you to work without lowering your head and curving your upper back. (Medieval monks and makers of Victorian schooldesks realized this!) You can buy a moulded perspex lectern-type stand called the Writing Slope,★ which is reasonably priced and well worth investigating. It's rather like a designer's drawing board, but transparent, so you can spot any papers that get shuffled under it.

If you do a great deal of copy typing or word-processing, you are probably painfully aware of discomfort in your back, neck and shoulders, caused by the unnatural position in which you have to hold your head as you continually look sideways and down at what you are copying. The Copyholder★ is a supported stand which holds your work upright, enabling you to look straight at it, reducing strain on the spine and on the neck and shoulder muscles.

If you can't accommodate a Copyholder, at least make sure that you alternate the sides on which you place the work to be copied, so that you are not always turning your head in the same direction. The side you are used to looking towards will always feel more 'natural' than the other side, so this will take a bit of discipline; but it will repay the effort, for if you habitually look to one side, you may develop more serious problems of the neck and spine.

I have used a Writing Slope and a Copyholder for several years, and have found them both extremely helpful.

Your lighting

Most offices are lit these days with fluorescent tubes, which provide basic overall illumination and are cheap to run. Some people find fluorescent lighting acceptable; for others it is unpleasant. If you don't like it, you might consider buying a desk lamp or two to provide softer, more direct light in your own office or corner. If your firm will not provide them, you may want to buy them yourself. You probably spend more of your time in your office than anywhere else, so a small investment in your comfort and well-being there isn't really an extravagance.

How you sit
When you sit properly, with your spine erect, your pelvis centred and the weight of your upper body supported by your pelvis, you are actually resting your body. Learning to sit well will do more for your comfort and overall well-being throughout your working day than anything else.

The structure of the body calls for sitting on the 'sitting bones' – the curved ridges of bone at the lower edge of the pelvis. When you do this, your pelvis is held in its upright, central position, and can support your spine, neck and head, and the whole weight of your upper body, as it is intended and designed to do.

When your pelvis is centred – as shown in the illustrations below – your spine can lift up from it, and lengthen instead of collapsing. The pressure on the vertebrae, especially the five lumbar vertebrae of the lower region of the spine, is reduced, and your entire spine is protected.

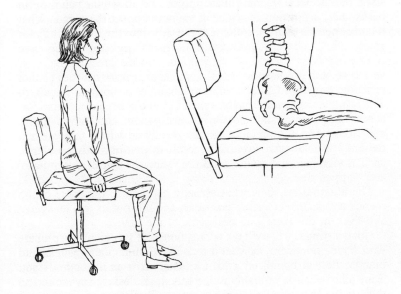

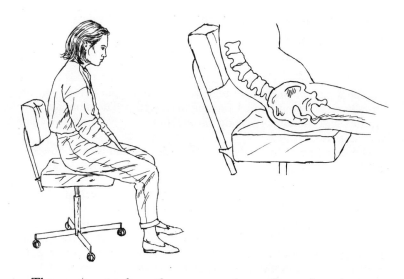

The common tendency, however – as shown above – is to slump: to sit on the coccyx at the base of the spine. This allows the pelvis to tilt backwards, a position in which it cannot support the spine. What then happens is that *you* collapse backwards into the support of your chair. This collapses your chest, constricting your lungs and restricting your breathing, as well as putting pressure on your vertebrae; and it squashes your abdominal organs so that they cannot function properly. Circulation throughout your body is impaired. The result is tiredness, irritability, inability to concentrate, muscular aches and pains; and possibly constipation and other minor afflictions. And the pressure on the vertebrae, which they are not designed to take, may eventually result in more serious problems, such as sacroiliac and sciatic conditions, and the so-called 'lumbago' and 'slipped disc'.

The illustrations show what actually happens to the spine in the correct and incorrect sitting positions, and most of us will recognize ourselves on this page – at least some of the time.

Good sitting starts with the sitting bones. If you aren't sure where your sitting bones are, or what it feels like to sit on them, you should practise first at home, on a firm kitchen chair or a wooden stool. Your office chair is probably well·padded, and I defy anyone to feel their sitting bones on a squashy surface. But once you experience correct sitting on a firm surface, you will be able to transfer that new sensation, and your new skill, to the office.

Here is how to assume the correct sitting position.

Sit towards the front of your chair. Place your feet flat on the floor, parallel and about hip width apart. Your knees should also be hip width apart, and a little lower than your hips. This will make it easier for you to maintain your pelvis in the central, upright position.

Slide your palms under your buttocks, and move your fingers until you feel two little rounded protuberances. These are your sitting bones.

Rock your trunk backwards and forwards on your sitting bones, tilting your pelvis to and fro and noting how the pressure on your fingers increases and lessens as you move. The point at which the pressure is greatest is the proper position for balancing the upper body on the sitting bones.

In this position your pelvis is central and upright. Your lower (lumbar) spine is nearer to the vertical, and will now be able to lift up from your pelvis.

Draw your shoulders up towards your ears. Then pull them gently back, squeezing your shoulder blades together. Then pull them down away from your ears and leave them there. Allow your arms to hang loosely by your sides.

Now begin to lengthen your spine. Start stretching gently up out of your pelvis, using the muscles of your back and not your shoulders. Feel that you are creating space between your hips and your ribcage, and between each and every one of your vertebrae. At the same time, feel that you are lengthening the front of your body: from your pubic bone to the top of your chest.

With your shoulders still pulled well down, tuck in your chin and lower your head, so that the back of your neck lengthens. Then slowly raise it, extending your neck without tensing it and directing the crown of your head upwards. Feel the space you are creating between your ears and your shoulders. Feel that you are being pulled gently up towards the ceiling by an invisible thread attached to the crown of your head at the top.

Check that your chin is level, parallel with the floor, neither pulled in nor jutting out. Your lips should be lightly closed, your teeth slightly open. Drop your jaw a little, and check on your tongue: if you find that it is clamped to the roof of your mouth, gently swallow and then let it remain at the bottom of your mouth, just behind your lower teeth.

Soften your gaze: don't stare, just gaze, and breathe steadily and evenly.

Now you are sitting well. Your pelvis is centred, supporting your spine which can lift up freely. Your chest is open, your ribcage is able to move freely, allowing your lungs to work properly. Your internal organs are being given plenty of space, which will help them to function optimally, aiding your circulation, digestion and elimination. Your whole body is poised, balanced, aligned, well-supported and, at the same time, relaxed.

This is a restful position for the body, for no undue strain is being placed on any part of its structure.

Sit in this way for a few minutes, observing your body and your posture, and the sensations of length, uprightness, balance and lightness. You may feel calmer, more alert, more clear-headed. Or, you may feel strange, different; or there may be a sense of strain in muscles unaccustomed to their new work. Just observe whatever it is you do feel, and be aware of it.

Observe your breath. Possibly you will find that it is slower, or deeper, or less constrained than before. Make no effort to control or to regulate it: again, just observe, don't judge.

Once you have got the feel of sitting well, practise it at work and at home whenever you think of it. In time, you will become increasingly aware of how you are sitting. You may become aware of strain when you slump, and how uncomfortable it really makes you, and will correct yourself whenever you catch yourself doing it.

At first, you may find correct sitting a strain. If you do, it is because your back muscles are relatively weak and not accustomed to supporting you in an upright position. What you are really aiming to do is to strengthen those muscles, so that you can rely on them, rather than on the back of your chair, to support you all the time! Eventually you will find it more restful to sit upright in this way. But be patient with yourself. If you have been collapsing all your life, your muscles *will* be weak, and will need strengthening. Correct sitting, combined with appropriate exercises, will bring this about, but it will take time. Meanwhile, when you do need to use your chair back for support, sit upright with the base of your spine right up against it – and don't feel guilty!

Vital though it is to sit well, it is equally important to avoid sitting in one position for too long. So try to move around as much as possible – consistent, of course, with getting your work done.

Do all you can to organize your work so that you can vary your tasks: don't stick at the same one for too long. Be crafty: find excuses for getting away from your desk. Learn to regard it as a temporary work-station, a place to which you come to do essential tasks, rather than a prison binding you hand and foot. Seek, rather than avoid, errands that take you out of your office. Go to see your colleagues in preference to ringing them up. Use the stairs instead of the lift. Stand up whenever you get the chance – for instance, while talking on the telephone, or sorting papers – to give yourself a change of position.

Sitting well will enhance your health and well-being, and will help you to avoid serious back problems and the various difficulties associated with restricted breathing. Once you develop the habit of sitting with an upright spine, not slumping your shoulders or collapsing your chest, you will probably find that you tire less easily, that you breathe more fully and deeply, and that the very uprightness of your posture makes you feel more alive, more responsive and more positive.

But the body needs movement, and suffers without it. In the chapters that follow we are going to look at what you can do throughout your day to ease muscles that have become tight and tense, and loosen joints that have become stiff, through too much sitting – and possibly even make such discomfort a thing of the past.

* The Labomatic chairs, the Writing Slope and the Copyholder are all available from Alternative Sitting, P.O. Box 19, Chipping Norton, Oxfordshire OX7 6NY (Telephone 0608 718875). They will supply information on these and other helpful products on request.

Chapter 2
The Exercises: Sitting

You probably regard exercise as something separate from your daily life, for which a special time has to be set aside at the beginning or the end of the day. And of course it is wonderful if you are able to build a good chunk of regular exercise - swimming, running, cycling, walking, or yoga practice – into your daily routine, either to get yourself off to a good morning's start, or to revive and renew yourself in the evening.

But if you also form the habit of integrating movement into your office life, you will be able to avoid the build-up of tension and strain during your hours of work.

In a traditional yoga class or home practice session, you would expect to go through a series of simple movements to prepare and loosen the joints and warm the muscles before going on to stronger work; and the session would normally include a balanced series of movements for the spine and the whole of the body. You would probably start, and certainly finish, with a period of relaxation.

In the office, what you will be doing is different. You'll be paying attention to how you feel throughout the day, and making a little bit of time here and there – a couple of minutes in every hour or so – to stretch yourself in whatever way you need to. No miracles of self-development or progress can be expected of this, but you *will* be able to release tension to a considerable degree, and to prevent it accumulating.

If you are alarmed at the thought of doing exercises in the office where people can see you, please don't worry. Many of the movements can be done quite unobtrusively, and you may grow bolder once you start feeling the benefit of what you are doing for yourself.

Everyone's working situation differs, and you will have to judge what is appropriate for yours. But you will find in this and the next two chapters enough to help you considerably, however formal or unsympathetic your working environment and/or your colleagues. If you work in a friendlier, less formal atmosphere, you will be able to do all the exercises. You will have a large repertoire of movements to choose from, according to how you are feeling and what you need at any given moment.

When you do the exercises, do them with as full awareness as possible. Try to take your mind off your work and absorb yourself fully in what you are doing. Even a minute or two spent like this will rest your mind as well as stretch your body, and you will return to your tasks refreshed.

Always work gently: never strain. Yoga is not about 'achievement': you aren't trying to 'get anywhere' or 'do' anything. You are *un*doing tension. Try to avoid involving muscles that don't need to be involved in a movement, so that you don't create additional, unnecessary tension.

If an exercise causes you pain or discomfort, that means that it is too strong for you, so you should leave it out. This applies to everything in the book, but particularly to the exercises for the neck and spine. Don't tolerate pain, thinking that 'if it hurts it must be good for you'. This isn't so. Pain is your body's way of telling you that what you are doing is *not* good for you. It is always a signal to stop. (This is probably even more important to remember in the office than it is in a class or home practice session, because you will be working muscles that are quite tense to start with.) This doesn't mean that you have to abandon that exercise forever: as you grow stronger and more supple, you may find that you can do things you couldn't manage a few weeks or months ago. The golden rule, always, is: listen to your body.

There are far too many exercises in this book for anyone to get through in one working day. What I hope you will do is work through the book and familiarize yourself with all of them, so that you will be able to call upon those that are likely to be most helpful to you as and when you need them. For example, if your neck and shoulders are your particular areas of tension, you will want to make frequent use of the exercises in this chapter. If you do a great deal of typing or writing or word-processing, you'll want to integrate the exercises for the fingers and hands, in Chapter 4, into your working day. If you spend a great deal of time looking at a computer screen, you will find the eye exercises, also in Chapter 4, useful – and so on. You'll want to do whatever is going to help you most at any given time, so the important thing is to be aware of how you are feeling, and take action when you need to, *before* your neck seizes up completely, or a tension headache starts.

If you enjoy the exercises, then of course you can do them at home, too, where you'll have more time. All of the exercises in Chapters 2, 3 and 4 can be done standing as well as sitting (except, possibly, for circling both ankles together). They can also be done sitting on the floor in a kneeling or cross-legged position, or with your legs straight out in front of you. The exercises for the toes, ankles, knees, hips, fingers, wrists and elbows (but not the shoulders) can also be done lying down.

The instructions for most of the exercises include directions for breathing. It is important that you follow them, for three reasons.

- Paying attention to your breathing will increase your awareness of what you are doing, and the more aware you are the more you will get out of the movements.

- Coordinating your movements with your breath will encourage fuller, deeper breathing.

- It will also bring your body and mind into harmony, so that even a few minutes' practice will leave you feeling mentally calmer and quieter, as well as physically better.

When no specific directions are given, breathe freely and naturally throughout the exercise. If you find yourself holding your breath, gently breathe out, and then carry on breathing normally.

All breathing should be through the nose, not the mouth.

The starting point for all the exercises in this chapter is the basic sitting position as described in Chapter 1.

Sit to the front of your chair, on your sitting bones, your feet flat on the floor and parallel, about hip distance apart. Place your feet a little in front of your knees, so that there is a nice, wide angle between your thighs and your lower legs. Pull your shoulders down away from your ears, and let your arms hang loosely by your sides. Lengthen your spine, and breathe freely.

Note: The exercises can all be done in normal daytime clothing, but for some you will need to loosen shirts or blouses that are tight at the neck or wrists.

THE SHOULDERS, NECK AND UPPER BACK

These are key tension collecting areas for most people. If you do a great deal of reading, writing, typing or word-processing, you will find that you can relieve the tension these activities cause, and avoid it building up, with the exercises in this section.

The neck is delicate, and should always be moved with care, particularly when it feels tight, tense and sore. It's best to start off with a few shoulder movements, to warm up the nearby muscles.

1 THE SHOULDERS

Shoulder circling

Sit in the basic sitting position, with your arms hanging loosely at your sides.Circle your shoulders gently forwards a few times, one at a time and then together. Then circle them gently backwards. Do this slowly, and enjoy it. Let your arms and hands be floppy.

Shoulder lifting and squeezing

Inhale and slowly lift your shoulders, drawing them up towards your ears.

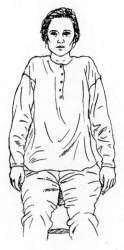

Exhale as you draw them back, squeezing your shoulder blades together. Pull back quite hard, as if you were trying to get your shoulder blades to meet in the middle.

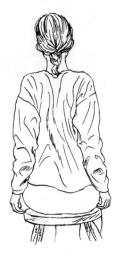

Continue to *exhale* as you draw your shoulders slowly but firmly down away from your ears, keeping them slightly back. Be aware of the space you are making between your ears and your shoulders. Imagine that a heavy suitcase in each of your hands is weighing you down.

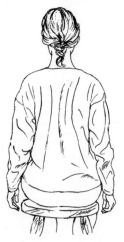

Repeat this as many times as you feel you need to. You will probably begin to feel a bit better after four or five.

Shoulder blade squeeze

Interlace your fingers behind you at seat level, elbows bent and arms relaxed.

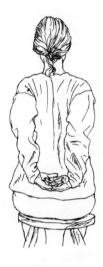

Exhale as you slowly draw your elbows towards each other, squeezing your shoulder blades firmly together.

Inhale as you release the squeeze.

Repeat this several times, working slowly and rhythmically, synchronizing movement with breath.

Arm rotations

Place your fingertips on your shoulders.

Inhale as you bring your elbows together in front of your chest, then lift them as high as possible, keeping them together for as long as possible. Direct them back, and then begin to lower them behind you.

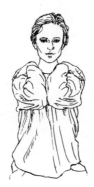
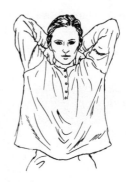

Exhale, squeezing your shoulder blades together, lowering your elbows as far as possible, and then bringing them forward and together.

Continue breathing and moving in this way, making the biggest possible circles with your elbows and coordinating movement with breath. Then reverse the direction of the movement, breathing in as you take your elbows back and up behind you; and out as you bring them down in front. Be aware that you are undoing tension throughout your entire upper body, especially your shoulders and upper back. You are also opening your chest and working your intercostal muscles (the muscles between the ribs that extend and contract the rib cage), encouraging fuller, deeper breathing.

This exercise is wonderfully invigorating. When you have done a few rounds of it, you will find your breathing stimulated, and your energy restored.

2   THE NECK

Head turning

This sequence is an adaptation of a yoga practice known as *Brahma Mudra*. It can be performed on its own or as a preliminary to the stronger stretches that follow. It will help to undo tension in your neck, calm your mind and aid your concentration. Perform the movements slowly and with awareness of what you are doing, synchronizing movement with breath. Let your eyes lead the movement, and let your head follow your eyes.

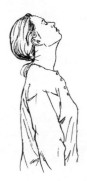 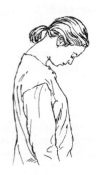

1
Inhale as you look forward, and then up towards the ceiling. Tip your head gently backwards, only as far as is comfortable.

Exhale as you slowly bring your head up and gently bend it forward, aiming your chin towards the notch in your throat.

Repeat twice more.

2
Exhale as you slowly look over your right shoulder, letting your eyes lead your head, keeping your chin level.

Inhale as you look to the front.

Exhale as you slowly look over your left shoulder.

Inhale as you look to the front.

Repeat twice more to each side.

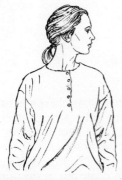

This sequence begins the process of gently stretching and lengthening the muscles of the neck and throat, and the upper back, without straining them. The next group of movements provides a series of stronger stretches for these muscle groups.

Stretching your neck: lowering head forwards

Establish your basic sitting position. Keep your shoulders relaxed as you lift up out of your pelvis, lengthening your spine. Allow your arms to hang loosely at your sides.

Exhale as you tuck in your chin and slowly lower your head, aiming your chin towards the notch in your throat. Hold this position, breathing freely, allowing your neck to lengthen and your head to grow heavier. You should feel a nice stretch through the back of your neck, possibly as far down as your shoulder blades.

If that feels comfortable, and you would like a stronger stretch, interlace your fingers behind your head, resting your palms gently on the knob at the back and allowing your elbows to drop forward on either side of your face. Don't tug at your head: you are simply using the gentle pressure of your hands and arms to increase the stretch. If this is too strong a stretch for you, take your hands away.

Hold your chosen position for a few moments, breathing freely, and feel that with each outbreath you are sinking a little further into the stretch. Allow your head, neck, arms, shoulders and spine to soften.

To come out of the stretch, breathe in as you slowly lift your head and lower your arms. Do a few shoulder circles backwards to finish.

This movement stretches the muscles of the neck and the upper back, relieving tension in this area.

Stretching your neck: lowering head sideways

Still sitting in the basic sitting position with your arms loosely by your sides:

Anchor your left hand under your chair seat beside you to avoid lifting your shoulder as you perform the movement.

Tuck in your chin slightly, and *exhale* as you gently lower your head sideways to the right, aiming your ear towards your shoulder. Breathe freely as you hold this position. You will feel a stretch along the left side of your neck, from the tip of your shoulder to the base of your ear.

For a stronger stretch, take your right hand up and over your head, and place it just above your left ear, keeping your elbow back. Remember not to tug at your head: the arm is there only to add weight and gently increase the stretch. Keep your left shoulder pulled well down away from your ear.

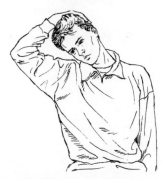

Hold this position, breathing naturally, allowing your head, neck, shoulders and arms to be soft; and feel that on each outbreath you are sinking more deeply into the stretch. Feel the length you are creating along the left side of your neck.

To come out of the stretch, lower your arm and then slowly lift your head on an inbreath.

Repeat on the other side. Then circle your shoulders backwards a few times.

Stretching your neck: lowering head diagonally

Sit in the basic sitting position, and anchor your left hand under your chair seat a little behind you.

Turn your head a quarter turn to the right, so that you face over your right knee.

Tuck in your chin, and *exhale* as you slowly lower your head towards your knee. You will feel a stretch somewhere between your left shoulder blade and the base of your skull on the left.

To increase the stretch, take your right hand up and over your head, and place it just above and behind your left ear, where the bone juts out. Your right elbow will be in line with your right knee.

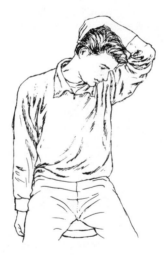

Hold this position, breathing freely, subsiding more deeply into the stretch on each outbreath.

To come out of the stretch, lower your arm and slowly lift your head, *inhaling*. Then turn to face front.

Repeat on the other side, and finish by circling your shoulders backwards a few times.

3 THE UPPER BACK

Because our eyes are in front and we are always looking forward, nearly all our movements are forward movements — reaching out to get things off shelves, reaching down to pick things up. In our daily lives we hardly ever need to make the compensatory movements that would bring the shoulders back into position, so the muscles that are meant to hold them back and down, and shape the upper back tend to lack tone, and we slump. The shoulders droop forward, the upper back rounds, and the chest collapses. All this has a negative effect on our breathing as well as on our posture, and maybe eventually even on our attitude to life in general. Working at a desk can easily accentuate all this. Sitting over our work, we feel fatigue, tension and possibly even pain between the shoulder blades. This can lead to irritability and depression. You will find the exercises in this section effective in relieving these conditions.

The chest expansion

Interlace your fingers behind your back. If you have enough room on either side of you, do this by moving your hands outward in a breast stroke movement: this will open the chest nicely and extend the ribcage, encouraging a full, deep breath.

Straighten your elbows, draw your clasped hands down towards your buttocks, and gently pull your shoulders back.

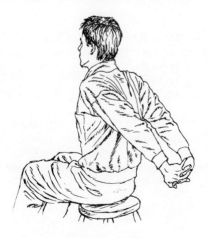

Inhale as you lift your arms away from your buttocks, keeping them straight. Lift them as high as you comfortably can, squeezing your shoulder blades together. You should feel a nice, strong squeeze.

Exhale as you lower your arms, allowing your elbows to bend.

Repeat a few times, working rhythmically with your breath. On your last repeat, hold the upper position for a few moments, breathing naturally. Then slowly lower your arms and release your hands on an outbreath.

Four upper back tension relievers

This sequence of four exercises is splendid for easing tension in the upper back, between the shoulder blades. It also gives a lovely stretch to the arms and the entire torso; and works the joints of the fingers, hands and wrists.

The sequence should be done in the order given, as the exercises increase in strength. If you want to do only one or two of them, do the first one or two. If you are doing them all, give your arms an occasional rest in between.

1
Sit in the basic sitting position. Interlace your fingers in front, turn your palms to face your knees, and *exhale* as you straighten your elbows.

Inhale as you push your palms away from you, raising your straight above your head with your palms facing the ceiling. Have a really good stretch upwards.

Make sure that you aren't tightening your jaw or neck.

Exhale and lower your arms to the front, continuing to stretch and push your palms away from you.

Repeat twice more, and then rest your hands in your lap.

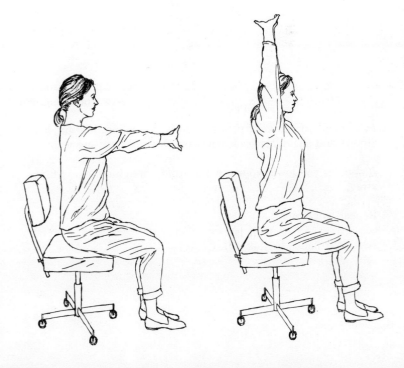

2

Interlace your fingers in front, turn your palms to face your knees and *exhale* as you straighten your elbows.

Inhale as you raise your straight arms above your head, palms facing the ceiling as in the previous exercise.

Exhale as you lower your clasped hands behind your head, turning your palms so they face the back of your head, but don't touch it. Direct your elbows and shoulders back, and feel the squeeze at the top of your shoulder blades.

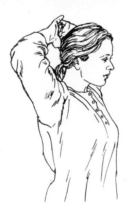

Inhale and stretch your palms towards the ceiling, keeping your elbows and shoulders back, and straightening your arms.

Exhale as you lower your arms in front, stretching your palms away.

Repeat twice more.

Rest your hands in your lap.

3

Interlace your fingers in front, turn your palms to face your knees and *exhale* as you straighten your elbows.

Inhale as you raise your straight arms above your head, palms facing the ceiling.

Exhale as you lower your clasped hands behind your head as in Exercise 2. This time, rest your cupped palms against the back of your head.

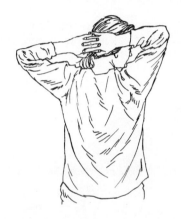

Keeping your elbows and shoulders well back, turn your head slowly to the right, and then to the left.

Repeat three or four more times to each side, breathing freely.

Inhale as you stretch your arms up, palms facing the ceiling.

Exhale as you lower your arms in front, stretching your palms away.

Rest your hands in your lap.

4

Interlace your fingers in front, turn your palms to face your knees and *exhale* as you straighten your elbows.

Inhale as you raise your straight arms above your head, palms facing the ceiling.

Exhale as you lower your clasped hands behind your head, keeping your elbows and shoulders back, and your hands a little away from your head.

Move your arms in large ovals behind your head, moving your elbows as far out to each side as possible, keeping them as low and as far back as possible. Do this three or four times, breathing freely; and then reverse directions.

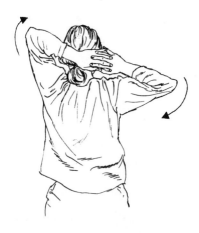

Inhale as you stretch your palms up towards the ceiling.

Exhale and lower your arms in front, stretching them and pushing your palms away.

Rest your hands in your lap.

Finish the sequence by gently circling your shoulders forwards and backwards a few times.

The Shoulder Blade Shove

This wonderful exercise works directly on the muscles of the upper back, toning, strengthening and increasing circulation to them. You may not get the feel of the movement right away because you aren't used to using these muscles, but if you persevere it will improve and maintain their tone, enabling you to improve your posture. It will also make you more aware of this area of your body, which, as you don't use it a great deal and cannot even reach it easily (for example, when scrubbing your back or doing up zips), may be a 'dead area' for you as it is for many people.

Sit in the basic sitting position with your arms loosely by your sides.

Lift your shoulders up, draw them back and gently pull them down away from your ears. Feel that your upper back is wide and flat, and your chest open.

Exhale and empty your lungs.

Inhale and slowly raise your arms sideways to shoulder level.

Exhale as you form your hands into loose fists with the thumbs curled outside.

Inhale as you slowly shove your shoulder blades and arms out, away from the midline of your body.

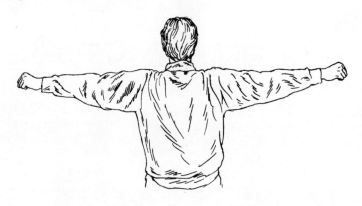

Think of the shoulder blade and the arm as forming a single unit. Feel that you are making space between the shoulder blades.

Exhale as you draw your shoulder blades together. Don't lift your shoulders or pull them back to do this: the work is all in the upper back.

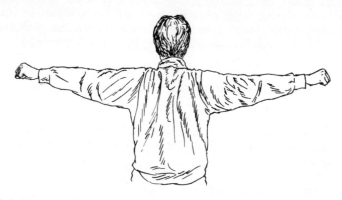

Inhale as you first stretch your fingers out and then bend your hands up at the wrists until your fingertips point towards the ceiling. Hold your shoulder blades firmly squeezed together as you do this.

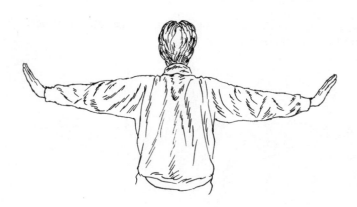

Exhale as you slowly lower your arms, keeping them straight, and squeezing your shoulder blades firmly together, until your arms are alongside your body.

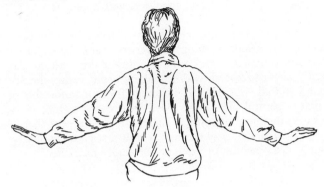

Then release the squeeze.

Repeat one to three more times, and gently circle your shoulders backwards a few times to finish.

The Shoulder Blade Shove is, for me, the ultimate exercise for 'reaching the parts that other exercises cannot reach'. In the long term, it will strengthen your spine and make it more flexible, and help you to correct or avoid round-shoulderedness. Meanwhile, you will find it a great help in relieving the five o'clock ache.

Tension-relieving massage

To end this chapter, here is a little massage you can give yourself to release tension in the neck and shoulders and upper back.

Place the palm of your right hand on your upper back on the left (if possible under your clothing) midway between the tip of your shoulder and your neck. Pick up a handful of skin and muscle, and gently begin to knead it, as if making bread, using the heel of your hand and all your fingers. This may feel uncomfortable or even slightly painful. The more tense you are, the tighter your muscles are, the more discomfort there will be. Respect that, and don't try to force your way through it, but just go on carefully massaging, not pinching or poking, but gently kneading.

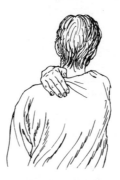

Then stop kneading, but keep holding your handful of skin and muscle. Gently shrug your shoulder up and down a few times. Then slowly and gently circle it backwards a few times.

Before massaging on the right side, slowly look over your left shoulder and then over your right shoulder. Notice the difference in how it feels and in how far you can see on each side.

Chapter 3
More Exercises: Sitting

THE SPINE

The spine is the vital centre of the body. It supports the head, and it enables us to maintain our upright stance. It encloses and protects the spinal cord and, with the brain, comprises the central nervous system which controls and regulates all the body's activities.

The spine consists of twenty-four vertebrae (five lumbar, twelve dorsal or thoracic, and seven cervical) plus the sacrum and the coccyx, and movement takes place at the joints between them. Potentially it is extremely mobile, but lack of movement and tightened muscles quickly cause it to stiffen and to lose its mobility and elasticity.

A stiff spinal column can lead to backache and more serious problems. Its restricted capacity for movement also hampers you in your daily activities and increases the risk of injury if you have a minor accident or lose your balance.

The spine is able to move in four directions: forwards, backwards, sideways and in rotation, and it should be moved regularly in all four ways.

The postures of classical yoga concentrate almost exclusively on the spine, and a balanced yoga class or practice session will always include examples of the four types of spinal movement. Although the classical yoga postures cannot be performed from a chair, there are many simple movements of each type which can.

The spine is an energy channel. For energy to flow freely through it, it needs to be maintained in a healthy, flexible condition, and it needs above all to be held erect. The exercises in this section will help you not only to relieve tension and tightness in the spine, but also to mobilize and strengthen it, so that you will find it easier to maintain the correct, balanced sitting posture. Practising them will also increase circulation to the spinal nerves, so that you will feel generally better, more energetic and alert.

Before you start to practise any of these exercises, establish your balanced sitting position. Make sure that you are sitting on your sitting bones, with your spine upright, long and aligned. In this way you will protect it from any possible injury.

Stretching the spine forwards

1
Sit in the basic sitting position.

Interlace your fingers in front and turn your palms to face your knees.

Inhale as you push your palms away from you, raising your straight arms above your head with your palms facing the ceiling. Stretch up out of your ribcage, lengthening the whole of your spine and the front of your body.

Exhale as you lean forward, stretching your palms away from you. The movement should come from your hips, and your spine, neck, head and arms should be in one long straight line, with your ears between your arms.

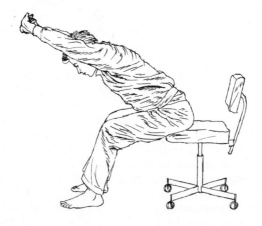

Inhale as you come back up, moving from your hips and stretching your spine. Stretch well up, pushing palms towards ceiling. Keep your pelvis tucked under to avoid arching your back.

Exhale as you slowly lower your arms to the front, and relax your hands in your lap.

Repeat once or twice more.

2

Sit in the basic sitting position with your chair well back from
your desk.

Place your feet about eighteen inches apart, flat on the floor and
parallel, a little in front of your knees. Rest your hands
comfortably on the tops of your thighs.

Exhale as you slowly fold forward from your hips, lengthening
your spine and keeping your head and neck in line with it. Allow
your hands to drop towards the floor and hang loosely. When you
have stretched as far forward as you comfortably can, gently lower
your head towards the floor and allow your back to round.

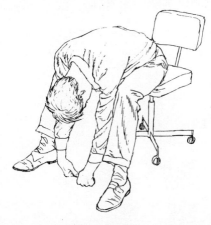

Hold this position, breathing slowly and deeply. Allow your hands
and arms to hang loosely and heavily, your neck free, your head
heavy. Feel that your whole upper body is letting go.

Inhale as you lift your head a little and slowly come back up,
maintaining the length in your spine.

This exercise not only stretches the spine, but gives the entire
upper body a chance to let go. It is an energizing exercise as well
as a very calming and restorative one.

Stretching the spine backwards

1
Sit in the basic sitting position and lengthen your spine.

Place your hands in the small of your back, thumbs pointing forwards.

Inhale and lengthen upward, lifting and opening your chest and your ribcage.

Exhale as you slowly stretch backwards in a smooth curve, continuing to lift your chest. Direct your shoulders back, and squeeze your shoulder blades together.

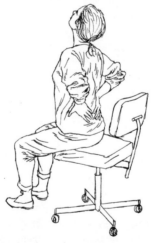

If this feels comfortable, slowly lower your head backwards, and look up at the ceiling.

Hold the position for a few moments, breathing naturally.

Inhale as you slowly come back to the upright position.

2

Sit in the basic sitting position.

Place the heels of your hands on the sides of your chair seat just behind you.

Inhale and lengthen up, lifting and opening your chest and ribcage.

Exhale and arch your upper back.

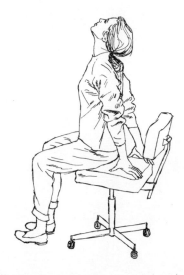

Draw your shoulders back and down, and gently bend your neck backwards, to look up at the ceiling.

Hold this position, breathing freely.

Inhale as you slowly come back to the starting position.

In these exercises, you need to make sure that you are working the upper back. It isn't important how far you go; what matters is that you work your whole spine, and do not overwork your lower spine. You should not feel any pressure in your lower back, but rather that your entire spine is stretching upward and curving backwards.

3

For this exercise, sit to the back of your chair, but be sure that your feet are still firmly planted flat on the floor. If they dangle, place some telephone directories or books, or an empty letter tray under them.

Interlace your fingers and turn your palms to face your knees.

Inhale as you stretch your arms forward and up, until your palms face the ceiling. Stretch up out of your ribcage.

Exhale as you stretch backwards over your chair back.

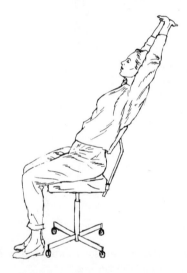

Hold the position for a few moments, breathing freely. Stretch on the inhalation, relax on the exhalation.

Inhale as you stretch your palms up towards the ceiling.

Exhale as you lower your arms to the front.

Stretching the spine sideways

In the side stretching exercises that follow, observe the following points:

- Your upper body should move as though between two sheets of plate glass at the front and back. The upper shoulder and hip shouldn't move forward.

- Your pelvis should be held firm and central so that your lower back does not arch.

- Your face should face forward, and your head should move in line with your body – no tucking in of the chin, or poking it out.

- Your abdomen should be held firm.

Both sides of your body should lengthen and curve smoothly: you should have no feeling of compression on the side you are stretching towards.

These three side-stretching exercises are a sequence: the gentlest first and the strongest last. It's best to do them as a sequence, but if you have time for only one, it should be the first one. There is always the danger of straining muscles by stretching too strongly when they are tight or cold.

1

Sit in the basic sitting position and lengthen your spine. Pull your shoulders down away from your ears and let your arms hang loosely by your sides.

Exhale as you slowly curve your upper body over to the right. Go only as far as you can without kinking at the waist: you are stretching, not bending, and both sides of your body should curve smoothly.

Let your right hand slide down, and your left hand up. Don't lift your left shoulder: keep it as relaxed as possible and down away from your left ear.

At the end of the outbreath, gently pull in on your lower abdominal muscles.

Inhale as you come slowly back up to the centre. In the centre, pause and lengthen upward.

Exhale as you slowly curve over to the left.

Inhale as you come up.

Repeat twice more to each side.

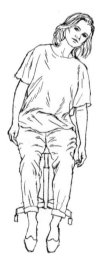

2

Sit in the basic sitting position, but place your feet a little more than hip width apart.

Inhale as you raise your arms sideways, bringing your fingertips together above the crown of your head. Leave your elbows comfortably bent so that your arms form a circle. Lengthen upwards, lifting your ribcage.

Exhale as you slowly curve over to the right, pulling in gently on your lower abdominal muscles. Lift your left elbow a little to increase the stretch along the left side of your body.

Inhale as you slowly come back up to the centre. Hold your abdomen firm, and do not arch your back.

In the upright position, centralize yourself and lengthen upwards.

Exhale as you slowly curve over to the left. This time lift your right elbow, increasing the stretch along the right side of your body.

Repeat twice more to each side.

Release your fingers and
finish by lowering your
arms to your sides,
exhaling.

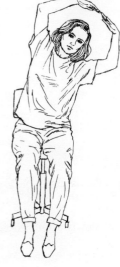

3

Sit in the basic sitting position.

Interlace your fingers in front and turn your palms to face your knees. Lengthen your spine.

Inhale as you push your palms away from you, raising your straight arms above your head with your palms facing the ceiling. Stretch yourself right up!

Exhale as you slowly stretch over to the right. Push your palms away, and feel the stretch along the left side of your body. Gently pull in on your lower abdominal muscles. Take care not to allow your left shoulder to drop forward.

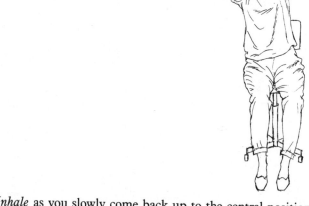

Inhale as you slowly come back up to the central position, and stretch up. Remember not to arch your lower back.

Exhale as you slowly stretch over to the left.

Repeat once or twice more to each side.

Stretch up, *inhaling*, and finish by lowering your arms to the front, *exhaling*.

Spinal rotations

The spine, as noted earlier, is capable of movement in four directions: forwards, backwards, sideways and in rotation. The exercises in this chapter have so far provided examples of the first three types of movement, and now we move on to the spinal rotations – more commonly referred to as 'twists'.

There are a great many ways in which the spine can be rotated. You can perform twisting movements from a standing position, or lying on the floor with the spine supported, or sitting on the floor, or – as in the exercises that follow – sitting in a chair.

However they are done, twisting movements have a beneficial effect on the spine, toning it and improving its mobility. They bring a rich supply of fresh blood to all spinal nerves and the muscles that support the spine, and are very energizing. They also help to redress the imbalances that come from over-working one side of the body, which office tasks such as writing, typing, word-processing and telephoning all tend to do.

Like the other spinal movements in this chapter, these are simple to perform, but certain precautions do need to be observed. Before you twist your spine, it is essential that it be upright and as long as possible, so that the vertebrae are free of compression. So first make sure that you are sitting really well, and take a few moments to monitor your position and lengthen your spine before you begin.

1

Cross your left arm over your body and place your palm against the outside of your right thigh. Take your right arm behind you and rest the back of the hand against your left waist.

Inhale as you lift up out of your pelvis, opening your chest and your ribcage.

Exhale as you slowly turn your head to look over your right shoulder. Let your eyes lead the movement: this will help to keep your neck nice and long.

Inhale and lengthen.

Exhale and twist your upper body around to the right, as far as you comfortably can. Allow your right shoulder to release and move backwards.

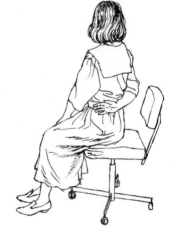

Hold this position, breathing slowly and calmly. With each outbreath, allow your body to move a little further into the twist. Don't force the movement, just allow it to take place.

Inhale as you slowly turn to face forwards. Then release your hands.

Repeat to the other side.

2
Sit in the basic sitting position.

Place your left palm against the outside of your right thigh. Place your right hand behind you and hold on to the back of your chair seat just below the base of your spine.

Inhale and stretch up, opening your chest and lifting your ribcage.

Exhale and slowly turn your head to the right, letting your eyes lead the movement, until you are looking over your right shoulder.

Inhale and lengthen your spine.

Exhale and twist your upper body around to the right, as far as you comfortably can, allowing your right shoulder to release backwards.

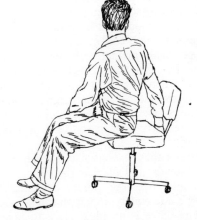

Hold the position, and breathe slowly and quietly, moving a little further into the twist on each outbreath. Do not force the movement: just allow it to happen as your breath flows.

Inhale as you slowly turn to face forwards. Then release your hands.

Repeat to the other side.

Chapter 4
More Exercises: Sitting

Most of the movements and postures of yoga are designed to work on the spine: to make it strong and flexible, and to promote the free flow of energy through it.

But although the spine is paramount, the other joints of the body shouldn't be neglected. This is especially true for people who do sedentary jobs, because sitting in one position for long periods tends, as we know, to stiffen the joints.

The exercises in this chapter systematically work all of the body's *other* joints – the fingers, hands, wrists and elbows (the shoulders were covered in Chapter 2); the toes, ankles, knees and hips. They are part of a group of yoga practices called *Pawanmuktasana*. This is a Sanskrit word which means 'wind-releasing', and it refers to the accumulation of toxins in the system.

Toxins build up due to a number of factors, including the ingestion of unhealthy foods and harmful chemicals; smoking and the consumption of alcohol, coffee, tea, sugar and salt; atmospheric pollution; and physical, mental and emotional stress. When the body is unable to deal with the toxins through the normal processes of elimination (i.e. when there is an excessive accumulation of them), they are thrown to the joints so as to safeguard the vital organs. The joints are therefore prime sites for the buildup of toxins, which cause stiffness and discomfort; and, in the case of arthritic conditions, pain and immobility.

Regular practice of these exercises for the joints can help to speed up the removal of toxins, and alleviate their effects. They also help to open, lengthen and free the joints, releasing them from the compression they are normally under, and to increase their mobility and strength. The office is an ideal place to practise them, since many of them, especially the ones for the feet and legs, can be done while you carry on with your work.

THE ARMS

Typing, word-processing and handwriting all involve the fingers, hands, wrists and elbows in very small, repetitive movements which result in strain, cramp and stiffness in these joints as well as creating tension in the neck and shoulders. They can also lead to painful conditions such as 'tennis elbow'. It is vital to give these joints different movements from time to time, to free them from cramp and strain, and to work the associated muscles.

Note: The directions for the exercises for the fingers, hands and wrists specify the arms to be held at shoulder height in front of you, but they can also be (more discreetly) practised with your arms and hands at your sides.

1 THE FINGERS AND HANDS

Stretching and squeezing

Sit in the basic sitting position.

Raise your arms to shoulder height in front, palms facing down. Focus your awareness in your fingers, and breathe naturally.

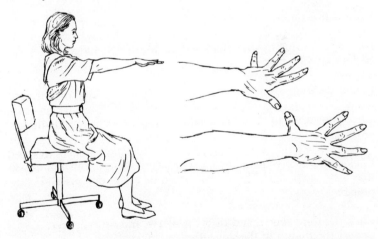

Open your hands slowly and stretch your fingers wide, making big spaces between each of your fingers, especially between the tips of your thumbs and little fingers. Feel the stretch across your palms.

Don't stiffen your fingers: feel that you are opening them and extending them, lengthening and creating space in them.

64

Now slowly curl your fingers, and make fists with the thumbs folded inside. Squeeze your thumbs, and gradually increase the strength of the squeeze as much as is comfortable.

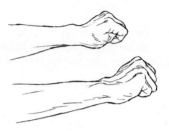

Carry on stretching and squeezing, making the movements smooth and fluid, not quick and jerky.

Keep your shoulders down and your spine lengthened, and remember not to tighten your jaw.

Do this five times.

Lower your arms to your sides and circle your shoulders backwards a few times.

Finger flicking

Raise your arms to shoulder height in front, your palms facing down.

Flick the tips of your index fingers sharply against your thumbs so that they 'snap' out. The action should be crisp, definite and precise.

Flick the third finger, and then the fourth and little fingers, against the thumb in the same way.

Then work back, flicking the fourth, third and index fingers.

Continue, gradually increasing the speed of the flicking, without losing the crispness and precision of the action.

Lower your arms and rest your hands in your lap.

Finger pulling

With your left hand, pull very gently along your right thumb. Do this several times. Then pull gently along your index, third, fourth and little fingers in the same way.

Then pull the fingers of your left hand.

Finger bending

Very gently bend your right thumb back towards your wrist with your left hand.

Then gently bend your index third, fourth and little fingers in turn.

Then gently bend the fingers of your left hand.

These two simple exercises are splendid for freeing the finger joints and releasing tension in them after you have been doing a lot of typing or writing. You should never overdo them, though: always do them very gently.

2   THE WRISTS

Wrist bending

Sit in the basic sitting position.

Raise your arms to shoulder height in front, your palms facing down.

Focus your awareness in your wrists, and breathe naturally.

Bend your hands backwards at the wrists, keeping your fingers straight and pointing them upward. Your palms face forward, as if pushing against a wall.

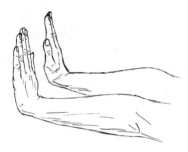

Slowly bend your hands forward at the wrists, pointing your fingers downward. Try to keep all three sets of knuckles straight: all the movement should be in the wrist joints.

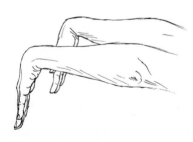

Repeat the movement five times.

Lower your arms and circle your shoulders backwards.

Wrist circling

Raise your arms to shoulder height in front, palms facing down.

Make a loose fist with your right hand, thumb inside.

Support your right elbow with your left hand, and circle your right fist slowly clockwise.

Make the circles as big as possible, working your wrist joint through its full range of movement.

Do this five times, and then reverse directions.

All the movement should be in the wrist: there should be none in the elbow or shoulder.

Repeat the exercise with the left wrist: five times in each direction.

Then repeat with both wrists, circling them together in the same direction, five times in each direction.

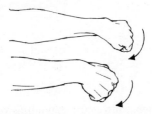

Lower your arms and circle your shoulders back.

Once you can isolate and control the movement in the wrist, keeping the rest of the arm still, it won't be necessary to support the arm.

Be aware of the 'quality' of the movement: whether it is smooth and 'well-oiled', or jerky and restricted. Be aware of the difference between your right and left wrists, and of any changes that take place as you practise over a period of time.

3 THE ELBOWS

Elbow bending: arms forward

Sit in the basic sitting position.

Raise your arms to shoulder height in front of you, with your palms facing up.

Focus your awareness in your elbows, and breathe naturally.

Exhale as you bend your elbows, bringing your fingertips to your shoulders, keeping your upper arms parallel to the floor.

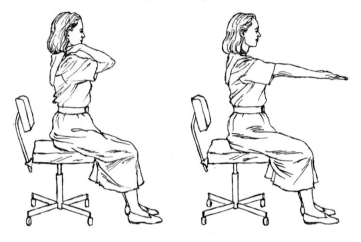

Inhale as you straighten your arms, extending your fingertips away. Do not 'lock' the elbows, wrists, or fingers, but feel that you are lengthening and opening all the joints. Feel that you are making space in your elbow joints.

Repeat five times.

Lower your arms and circle your shoulders back.

Elbow bending: arms to the sides

Raise your arms sideways to shoulder height, palms facing up.

Exhale as you bend your elbows, bringing your fingertips to your shoulders, keeping your upper arms parallel to the floor.

Inhale as you straighten your right arm, extending your fingertips away, lengthening and opening the elbow joint.

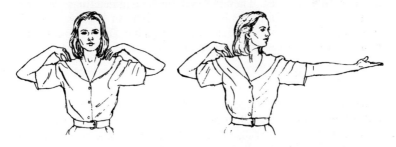

At the same time, letting your eyes lead the movement, turn your head slowly to the right.

Exhale as you return your fingertips to your shoulders, simultaneously turning your head to look forward.

Inhale as you straighten your left arm, turning your head to the left.

Exhale as you return your fingertips to your shoulders, turning your head to look forward.

This is one round. Do two more.

Lower your arms and circle your shoulders back

Throughout these two exercises, keep your shoulders down and your spine lengthened, and remember not to tighten your jaw.

THE LEGS

Sitting for long periods not only stiffens the joints, but tends also to make the circulation sluggish, pooling the blood in the feet and the lower legs. Exercising the feet and ankles not only increases mobility of the joints, but also helps the muscles to assist the veins in pumping the blood back up the legs, against the force of gravity, to the heart.

The following exercises can be done at almost any time while you get on with your work. They can even be done in meetings – but you do need to be careful not to lose track of whatever is going on in the meeting (and also not to kick your Managing Director under the table, as I have occasionally been known to do).

1 THE TOES

Poor toes! They work so hard for us, supporting us day in and day out as we stand and walk around; and they are so crucial to our balance and to our carriage. Yet we forget them, and neglect them. Perhaps this is because they are so far away from our head.

Toe exercises are important, and doing them makes you feel better all over.

Toe bending

If possible, remove your shoes and socks (or at least your shoes). Your feet will be glad to be exposed to the air, and they will stretch better too.

Sit in the basic sitting position with your feet flat on the floor, hip width apart.

Lift your right foot and straighten the leg in front.

Focus your awareness in your toes, and breathe naturally.

Gently push your heel away from you, and draw your toes back towards your body. You should feel a slight stretch along the back of your leg.

Slowly curl your toes forward. There should be movement at both sets of toe joints, but none at the ankle: the foot remains upright.

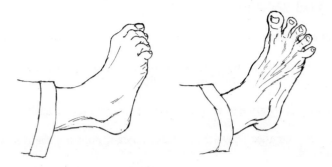

Don't curl so tightly that you get cramp.

Straighten your toes and bend them back towards you. At the same time, spread them, pulling your big toe as far away from your little toe as possible. Try to make space between each and every toe.

Repeat five times, and then do your left toes.

This exercise, and the following ones for the ankles, can also be done:

● with the heels on the floor

● standing up (while waiting for your bus or train)

● sitting on the floor with your legs outstretched in front (perhaps while watching television at home)

● lying down (for a wake-up stretch in the morning, or if you are ill in bed).

2 THE ANKLES

Ankle bending

Sit in the basic sitting position and straighten your right leg in front, the left foot still flat on the floor.

Focus your awareness in your ankle, and breathe naturally.

Stretch your toes forward as far as you can, pointing them away from you.

Then push your heel away from you, bringing your toes back towards your body. Feel the stretch along the back of your leg, from the heel to the buttock.

Do this five times, slowly. Repeat on the left.

Your leg should remain straight throughout, and all the movement should be in the ankle: there should be none at the hip or knee.

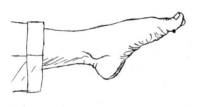
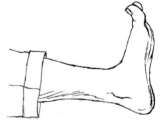

Ankle circling

Sit as before and straighten your right leg in front, the left foot flat on the floor.

Push your heel away, so that you feel the pull along the back of your leg.

Slowly circle your right foot clockwise and then anti-clockwise, five times in each direction. Make the circles as big as possible so that you work your ankle joint through its full range of movement.

You can imagine you are drawing circles with a compass: your ankle is the fixed central point, and there is a pencil at the end of your big toe. Draw the circles bigger and bigger.

Repeat on the left.

Keep your shoulders down and your spine lengthened. There should be no movement at the knee or hip, only at the ankle.

Be aware of the 'quality' of the movement: whether it is smooth and 'well-oiled', or jerky and crunchy. Be aware of the difference between your right and left ankles. Be aware of any changes that take place as you practise over a period of time.

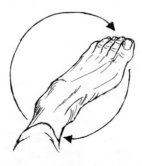

3 THE KNEES

Knee bending

Sit to the back of your chair, your feet flat on the floor and parallel, hip width apart.

Focus your awareness in your knees, and breathe naturally.

Raise and straighten your right leg, pushing your heel gently away, and then bend it fully.

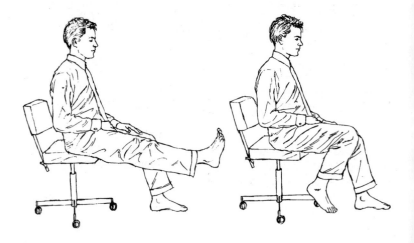

Repeat five times.

Repeat on the left.

Knee circling

Sit in the basic sitting position, feet flat on the floor and parallel, hip width apart.

Focus your awareness in your knees, and breathe naturally.

Raise your right leg and circle it clockwise and then anti-clockwise. The foot dangles loosely, and the movement is at the knee.

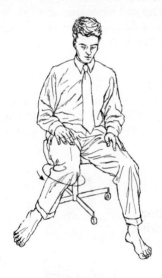

Repeat five times in each direction.

Repeat on the left.

THE HIPS

Next to the shoulder, the hip is the most mobile joint of the body. But it needs movement to remain mobile, and suffers particularly badly from our habit of sitting in chairs for extended periods.

The best thing you can do for your hip joints is to be active. Get plenty of exercise: walking and swimming are both excellent. When walking, lengthen your normal stride by just one inch: this is an effective way of working on these joints.

In the office, get up and move around as much as you can. There is a limit to what can be done in your chair to exercise your hip joints, but here are two suggestions:

1
Sit in the basic sitting position.
Place your right ankle on your left thigh, just above the knee.
Relax your right leg, allow your knee to drop towards the floor, and let gravity and the weight of your leg gently open out your hip joint.

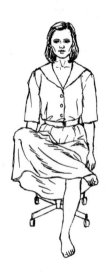

This is a passive stretch. You don't need to do anything: just sit like this for as long as is comfortable while you get on with your work. Change legs carefully after five minutes or so.

2
If you are fairly loose in the hips, and if you are wearing suitable clothing, and if your chair is suitable, you may find that you can comfortably sit cross-legged on your chair seat.

Or, bring the soles of your feet together on your chair seat, your heels as close as possible to your buttocks.

Both these exercises are good for opening out the hips, and if they are not feasible for you at work, you could practise them at home (while you are watching television, perhaps: see Chapter 7).

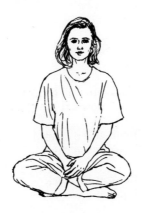

THE EYES

The eyes are muscle, too; and they also get strained, tired and tense in the course of the working day. Often, when we are concentrating on our work, we tend to stare at it, which is very wearing for the eyes. Be aware of this, and as much as possible, keep your gaze gentle, and close your eyes for a few moments now and then to rest them.

Eye exercises will relax, revitalize and strengthen your eyes. Here are two very simple ones.

Watching the clock

Close your eyes, and imagine that you are gazing at the face of a huge clock (with numbers and hands, assuming you are old enough to remember pre-digital days). Imagine the clock face filling the entire wall in front of you. Then open your eyes.

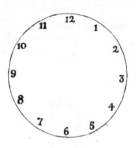

Look up at 12 o'clock
Look down at 6 o'clock

Look at 3 o'clock
Look at 9 o'clock

Look at 1 o'clock
Look at 7 o'clock

Look at 2 o'clock
Look at 8 o'clock

Look at 11 o'clock
Look at 5 o'clock

Look at 10 o'clock
Look at 4 o'clock

Repeat each of these several times before going on to the next.

Finally, move your eyes slowly round in big, smooth circles, starting at 12 o'clock and working right round the clock face. Do this a few times in each direction.

Palming

When you have been doing a great deal of 'close' work, and your eyes feel as though they just can't take any more, give them this treat, which only takes a minute or two.

Rub the palms of your hands very briskly and energetically together. When you've got them really warm and tingling, place them over your closed eyes and sit quietly for a few minutes, holding them gently, not pressing the eyes. Feel that the warmth and energy from your hands – your own healing energy – is being transmitted to your eyes, soothing, relaxing and refreshing them.

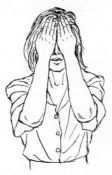

Breathe softly, surrendering each outbreath with a long, gentle sigh.

Let go. Just allow your eyes to be completely passive, and to take what they are being given.

Open your eyes behind your hands and gaze softly into darkness.

Finally, slide your fingertips softly down along your forehead, your eyelids, your nose, your cheeks, your lips and your chin.

AND FINALLY...

Nothing is more draining, or more tiring, than the way in which we dissipate energy by trying to do and to think about more than one thing at a time. You should really try to do just one thing, and give your full attention to it. This is a counsel of perfection: in most jobs, there are so many conflicting demands on your time and energy that it can be difficult to concentrate, and you end up trying to do three or ten things at once. Then the phone goes, and you have to drop everything and deal with whatever crisis it has announced. And so it goes on...At such times, it helps just to drop everything for a few moments, and stop.

So the sitting exercises end with an exercise that is just that: sitting. And, of course, breathing.

Sit in the basic sitting position and rest your hands comfortably in your lap: lightly clasped, folded, or palms down on your thighs. Begin to focus your awareness on your breath, and watch each inbreath and each outbreath.

When it feels natural to do so, blink slowly once or twice and then gently close your eyes.

Observe your breath. Observe it entering and leaving your nostrils. Observe its passage up and down your nostrils. Observe its temperature and its texture.

Don't attempt to control or regulate your breath: don't do anything to change it. Just observe your own natural breath.

Let your outbreath take its course: let it take as long as it needs to leave your body. Let there be a little space between each outbreath and the next inbreath. In that little space, just be still.

Continue breathing in this way for a few minutes, and then gradually begin to increase the depth of your breath. Gently stretch your fingers and hands, and slowly open your eyes.

By focusing your awareness on your breath, you concentrate energy. This practice clears and calms your mind, roping in your scattered forces so that you can then decide what you are going to do next, and give your full attention to it.

Chapter 5
Breathing

Life is breath and breath is life. So long as there is breath in the body there is life.

Kaushitaki Upanishad

There is a saying: 'He who only half breathes, only half lives'. The way that we breathe affects the quality of our lives at every moment: not only our physical health, but our emotional stability and our mental balance. Faulty breathing is at the root of many illnesses; and is also a cause of that habitual, half-alive state of droopiness and lethargy that so many people unfortunately regard as normal.

Good breathing is full, deep, slow and rhythmic, and has many benefits.

- It helps to release tension.

- It helps to overcome fatigue and to replenish energy.

- It calms the mind, the nerves and the emotions.

- It improves sleep.

- It improves memory, concentration and all mental processes.

- It purifies the blood by supplying more oxygen for the body cells.

When you breathe really well, utilizing the full capacity of your lungs, your respiratory system functions at its best. As a result, your circulation, digestion and elimination improve. You feel physically better, and this can transform your state of mind. In fact, it is true to say that the good functioning of all the body systems, and thus the quality of your entire life, depends upon the quality of your breathing.

You breathe in order to absorb oxygen, which is needed by every cell in the body for the activities of life to be carried on; and to discard carbon dioxide, the waste product of those activities. When you breathe in, oxygen is drawn from the atmosphere into the lungs and thence to the blood which, pumped by the heart, carries it around your body. When you breathe out, you throw off the carbon dioxide collected by the blood from all the body's tissues.

The lungs are elastic, flexible and capable of enormous expansion. If they were opened up and spread out, they would cover an area about forty times as large as the skin of the whole body. Their capacity is huge, but few people utilize more than a fraction of it.

When you are asked to 'take a deep breath', it's likely that you lift your upper chest and thrust it out, possibly accompanying this action with a loud sniff or a gasp. This doesn't help you to breathe more deeply: indeed, it nearly always has the reverse effect, because it actually reduces rather than increases the space within your chest cavity, and this compresses the lungs instead of enabling them to expand.

Your lungs can in fact be compared to a pair of balloons: when inflated, they are able to expand in all directions: forwards and backwards, out to the sides and downwards, as well as upwards. Whether or not they actually do so depends upon the tone and elasticity of the muscles involved in the breathing process: principally the intercostal muscles and the diaphragm, but also, to some extent, the abdominal muscles.

Breathing is controlled by nerve impulses sent by the brain, via the nerves, to the intercostal muscles and the diaphragm. These impulses are not under our conscious control, and the muscular action they initiate is automatic. What *is* under our conscious control is the condition of the muscles and the quality of their action, which we can improve, thereby improving the quality of our breathing.

Let us briefly examine the muscles involved in the breathing process, and the role played by each of them.

1   The intercostal muscles

The intercostal muscles occupy the spaces between the ribs, and their function is to extend and contract the ribcage to allow full inhalation and exhalation to take place.

The action of the ribs when the intercostal muscles are working properly is smooth and free, and can be compared to that of a bucket handle. Remembering that they are attached to your spine at the back and to your breastbone in front, you can visualize that 'bucket handle' action: as you breathe in they swing upwards and outwards towards the armpits, enlarging the space within the chest so that the lungs can expand and fill. As you breathe out they relax back down to their original position. The space within the chest is reduced, and the lungs return to their resting state.

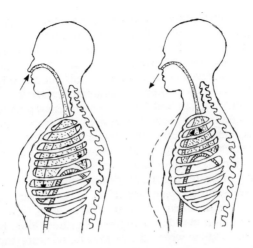

2 The diaphragm

The diaphragm is a large, strong, dome-shaped sheet of muscle separating the chest and abdomen. Along with the intercostal muscles, its function is to alter the dimensions of the space within the chest, allowing the lungs to expand and fill, subside and empty. As you breathe in your diaphragm moves downwards, playing its part in increasing the space within the chest cavity. As you breathe out it relaxes and returns to its resting position, and the space within the chest is reduced.

Although the action of the diaphragm is automatic, as explained earlier, the *quality* of its action is related to the condition of the intercostal muscles. If their tone is poor and there is little movement, the action of the diaphragm will be correspondingly limited. When both are functioning well, the movement of the diaphragm is unrestricted and pronounced, and breathing is slow, full and rhythmic.

The movement of the diaphragm also helps to massage, exercise and tone the abdominal organs.

3 The abdominal muscles

The abdominal muscles also have a role to play in the breathing process. The diaphragm, placed as it is between the chest and abdomen, forms the floor of the one and the roof of the other. When it moves downwards on an inbreath to enlarge the space within the chest, the room for it to do so has to be made in the abdomen below. The abdominal muscles create this space by moving slightly forwards. On the outbreath both the diaphragm and the abdominal muscles relax and return to their resting positions.

During a normal inbreath the abdomen should remain relaxed. Pushing it forwards deliberately, as some books and teaching methods used to advise, will result in forced, unnatural breathing. It will also distend and weaken the abdominal muscles, so you may develop a pot belly as well! However, a slight pulling in of the abdominal muscles towards the end of an outbreath assists the upward movement of the diaphragm and encourages a more complete exhalation. More residual air is expelled from the lungs, and the abdominal organs are massaged. This is also the most effective way of exercising the abdominal muscles.

This is a very basic explanation of the muscular activity that takes place when you breathe. You don't need an intellectual understanding of it in order to improve your breathing; but it can be quite helpful to know where the various muscles are and what they do, so that you can visualize their action.

If you are asking yourself whether or not you need improve your breathing, the answer is, almost certainly, 'Yes'. Very few people breathe well. Babies and young children do, but most of us lose the ability as we grow older. Poor postural habits, poor eating habits, stress, tension, emotional problems, lack of exercise, atmospheric pollution, smoking, all contribute to restricted breathing, i.e. breathing that is shallow, rapid and irregular; taking place mainly in the upper chest with little use of the ribcage; and correspondingly little use of lung capacity.

As such a pattern of restricted breathing develops in an individual, less and less work is demanded of the intercostal muscles. They forget what they are supposed to be doing, and lose their natural elasticity and resilience. The ribcage becomes fixed, the action of the diaphragm is restricted, and quick, shallow breathing comes to seem normal. Everything suffers.

Changing faulty breathing habits is very largely a matter of restoring tone and elasticity to the intercostal muscles so that they can start doing their job properly again. The way *not* to set about this is suddenly to decide that you are going to breath more deeply from now on: this will only result in a forced way of breathing that will feel unnatural and make you uncomfortable.

The best way to start developing healthier breathing habits is to exercise, which increases your need for oxygen and makes your breathing apparatus work more efficiently. Most forms of exercise – walking, running, swimming, cycling etc – will help. But even while sitting or standing you can practise exercises specifically designed to work the intercostal muscles; so that the ribcage extends, the chest opens, and the lungs expand. When all these things are happening, your breath will deepen and slow down automatically.

The breathing habits of a lifetime cannot be changed overnight, but if you practise regularly – even if only for five or ten minutes a day – you will soon begin to observe changes. As the tone of your intercostal muscles improves, a more efficient breathing pattern will take over naturally, increasing the flow of energy throughout your entire system, improving your concentration as well as your physical health, and fostering a heightened sense of well-being.

Many of the exercises already described in this book work in this way: especially the arm rotations, the upper back exercises, the chest expansion, and the various spinal stretches. And in the next chapter you will find directions for several movement and breathing sequences which are done from a standing position, and which are particularly helpful for developing better breathing habits.

It has to be said that office life offers very little encouragement to better breathing. You are sitting indoors without fresh air; and you get very little of the exercise that would increase your body's need for oxygen and put your lungs and all your breathing muscles to work. Sitting badly (if you do) makes matters worse: if your spine is slumped, your chest collapsed and your abdomen squashed, you are not going to be able to breathe properly!

As always, the important thing is to sit well. Breathing is something you do all the time, after all, and you need to create suitable conditions for this vital activity. When sitting, this means maintaining an upright, relaxed posture: a straight and lengthened spine and an open chest, which will give your ribcage space and freedom to move, and your lungs room to expand. Correct sitting is explained in Chapter 1. If you learn to sit well, you will be giving yourself a chance to breathe well all the time.

When you are practising the exercises in this book, I hope you will observe the instructions given for breathing, and try to establish a smooth, harmonious coordination of your movement and your breath. This coordination of movement and breath lies at the heart of yoga. More than anything else, it is what makes yoga different from other systems of movement, and so much more than just exercise.

Yoga is a Sanskrit word, and it means *union*. This can be explained in several ways, but at the most basic level, yoga is the union – the coordination – of body, mind and breath. Yoga aims to bring about balance, harmony and integration in the individual. Coordination of movement and breath, and breath awareness, are central to this process. They are, in fact, the keynote of all yoga practice.

The breath is the vital link between the body and the mind. We practise breath awareness and breath coordination with the aim of bringing body and mind into harmony. By observing and following the breath we harness energy, so that we can conserve rather than squander it; channel rather than dissipate it. Through breath awareness we begin to establish 'one-pointedness', or concentration – that state of mind which is not only the starting point for all meditational practices, but also necessary for our full functioning as human beings, able to fulfil our responsibilities and our potential.

In a yoga class, you would expect to spend an hour or more practising a balanced series of movements and postures, coordinated with the breath. A session usually begins, and always finishes, with a short period of relaxation. The practice of breath awareness, maintained throughout the session, calms, steadies and focuses the mind, so that through your practice of postures and breathing, your awareness is deepened. You are helped to turn your attention inwards, so that you grow more sensitive to your inner being. This may lead, in the concluding relaxation, to a sense of profound stillness, refreshment and peace: of oneness with your inner self. In time this sense of oneness and wholeness may become an abiding feature of your experience, and it may broaden out to a corresponding sense of unity with all of life and creation.

The concentrated atmosphere of a well-taught class, or the peace and quiet of your own home, are naturally more conducive than the work environment to attaining this state of harmony. But the principle is the same, whether you are practising for two hours or two minutes.

With regular practice you may find, even at work, that you grow increasingly able to drop your concern with the problems on your desk for a few moments; tune in to yourself, and absorb yourself wholly in what you are doing.

You may also find, after a while, that you derive so much pleasure and benefit from the exercises that you want give more time to them, and start to practise at home. If this happens for you, your practice may bear fruits that you did not anticipate; and what began with the specific hope of relieving specific tensions will become an integral and vital part of your life, nourishing and transforming it.

And what is the life breath? It is pure consciousness. And what is pure consciousness? It is the life breath. Kaushitaki Upanishad

Chapter 6
The Exercises: Standing

The movements and sequences in this chapter are all designed to encourage deeper, slower, more rhythmic breathing by improving the tone and strength of the intercostal muscles. Unlike the exercises in the earlier chapters, which can all be done sitting in your chair – 'on the job', as it were – these are to be performed from a standing position.

Of course these standing exercises aren't quite as inconspicuous as the sitting ones. I hope that it will be possible for you to do at least some of them in the office, but if circumstances make this difficult for you, perhaps you will be able to practise them at home.

Think: is there somewhere in your building where you can go to be alone for a few minutes, like a rest room, an unused meeting room, or even a loo? If there is, you will be able to retreat now and then. If not, are there 'quiet times', times when everyone else is in a meeting or gone to lunch?

Provided you can find yourself a space, or a quiet moment, you will be able to use the movements and sequences in this chapter. They will wake you up and get you going again if you are flagging, or calm you down and focus your mind if you have got a bit frantic. They will all help to balance your energies.

All the exercises and sequences start from the basic, balanced standing position. You will need a bit of time to practise learning to stand well, and I suggest that you do this at home. Then you will be able to establish the basic standing position fairly quickly in your little sessions at work.

Getting the position of the pelvis right is the key to standing well, just as it is to sitting well. As in sitting, it needs to be held centrally so that the spine can lengthen up from it. But whereas in sitting, the problem is that the pelvis is usually tipped backward so that the spine curves out and collapses backward; in standing what tends to happen is that the pelvis tips forward. This creates an exaggerated hollow in the small of the back, which compresses the vertebrae and prevents the spine from lengthening.

The continual pressure on the vertebrae, intensified by the downward pull of gravity, squeezes and flattens the cushioning matter – the discs – between them. The problem is compounded by lack of movement; and by the aging process, which brings its own deterioration, although this can be slowed down to a considerable degree by correct posture and correct movement. Eventually, some quite normal, inoffensive activity like gardening, or bending down to take a dish out of the oven, precipitates the extreme pain of the so-called 'slipped' (more accurately called prolapsed) disc, which appears to strike out of the blue, but is usually the result of strain and pressure over a long period of time.

You can see how important it is to hold the pelvis correctly. It is the very centre of balance in the body, and all the other parts of the body are connected to it. It supports the spine and the whole of the upper body, but it cannot do this well if it is not held centrally. In turn, the legs support the pelvis, but cannot do so properly if it is incorrectly placed.

Learn how to position your pelvis correctly by means of the excellent exercise that follows.

The Pelvic Tilt

Stand with your feet hip width apart, and parallel.

Place your right hand just below your waist in front, fingertips pointing down towards your pubic bone, and your left hand at the back, pointing down towards your tailbone.

Exhale as you squeeze your buttocks together and draw them down and in, tucking your pelvis under you. Feel with your hands how your pubic bone tilts up towards your face, and your pelvis at the back moves down and under. Feel how your lower abdominal muscles draw in, allowing the front of your body to lengthen. This is the correct position for your pelvis to be in.

Inhale and gently tilt the pelvis the other way, slightly arching your back. Note the increasing hollow in the small of your back as the top of your pelvis tips forward.

Repeat this movement slowly, several times, so you get to feel the difference between the two positions.

Now try it another way. Place your hands on your hip bones as you do the same movements. Feel how your hip bones at the top of your pelvis move forward and back.

Practise this several times, being aware of everything that is happening. You are learning to sense the correct, central position of your pelvis. If you are accustomed, as so many people are, to over-arching your lower back, the correct position will feel strange to you at first. But persevere: the lifelong health of your spine depends upon learning to stand well.

(**Note:** Although this problem is very common, not everyone has it. Occasionally the opposite occurs, and then it is necessary to learn to tilt the pelvis the other way.)

Another advantage of learning to position your pelvis correctly is that when it is held centrally it will do the job it is meant to do of holding your abdominal contents in place. Imagine the floor of your pelvis as a wide, shallow bowl, holding a large helping of spaghetti. When you stand with your lower back arched and the top of your pelvis tipped forward, it all spills over the rim! Quite apart from how this looks, it interferes with the functioning of the digestive and eliminative processes, and is not a good thing for the female reproductive organs.

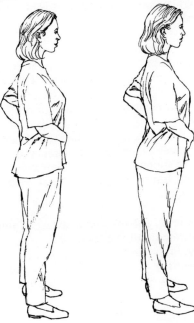

Standing

Once you have got the feel of centring your pelvis, you will discover a whole new dimension to standing – which, although it seems a very simple thing to do, is actually a very subtle and complex process.

Stand with your feet parallel and hip width apart, so that your feet come directly under your hips.

Lift your shoulders up, pull them back, and then draw them down away from your ears. Allow your arms to hang loosely at your sides.

Breathe naturally.

Make sure that your tongue isn't clamped to the roof of your mouth, but resting loosely in the bottom of it, behind your lower teeth, so that your jaw and throat soften.

Soften your gaze: don't stare. Continue to breathe steadily. If you find yourself holding your breath, exhale gently and then continue breathing naturally.

Now squeeze your buttocks together and tuck your pelvis under you – as if you had a tail and were drawing it down between your legs with a little tucking-under movement. This will bring your pelvis central, allowing your legs and thighs to lift up freely towards it, and your spine to stretch up out of it.

As you perform this 'tucking' movement, feel how your abdomen flattens and lengthens as the lower abdominal muscles begin to work, holding and supporting the abdominal contents, working together with your buttocks and your lower back muscles to support your trunk.

Take your attention to the soles of your feet. The weight should feel evenly distributed on them: take time to make any adjustment that is necessary. Press the balls of your feet into the ground, and feel your arches lifting.

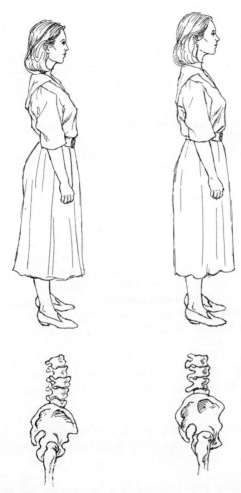

Left: Incorrect standing position: lower back over-arched, pelvis tipped forwards.

Right: Corrected standing position: pelvis centred, spine lengthened.

Now gently begin to lift the muscles of the insides of your legs. Pull gently up on your kneecaps, using the muscles at the front of your thighs. Don't push your knees back aggressively, or 'lock' them: the backs of your knees should feel soft. Feel how your thighs and buttocks are supporting your pelvis. Feel your pelvis very well centred.

Now begin to lift up out of your pelvis, lengthening your spine upwards and keeping your shoulders down. (Your shoulders, arms and hands are not involved at all in what you are doing, so don't try to 'hoik' yourself up with them.)

Feel that you are creating space between your hips and your ribcage. At the same time feel that you are lengthening up through the front of the body: from your pubic bone to the top of your chest.

Without lifting your chin or tensing your jaw, direct the crown of your head towards the ceiling. Feel that your neck is lengthening, and that space is being created between your ears and your shoulders. Imagine that you are being pulled up towards the ceiling by an invisible thread attached to the crown of your head.

Your chin should be level with the floor, not jutting out or pulling in. Check this, and gently move your head from side to side a few times to ensure that your neck is free, and that you haven't tightened it or your jaw.

Close your eyes and breathe steadily. Observe yourself and be aware of your whole body: lifted, lengthened, balanced and aligned.

All the classical yoga postures have Sanskrit names, and the name of this one is *Tadasana*. It means 'The Mountain Posture', and when you do it you can think of a mountain and all its qualities: strength, stability, uprightness, beauty and grandeur. You can also think of how the mountain, although firmly rooted in the ground, aspires upwards; and use this as a visualisation, or metaphor, for your own life and what you want to be or to achieve.

Tadasana is one of the most important of all the yoga postures, both in itself, and because it forms the basis of all other standing postures and movements. It is also one of the easiest to practise, because you can always find time and space for it. Practise it while waiting for your bus or train, or in the supermarket queue, or at the photocopier.

Pay attention to how you stand throughout all your daily activities that involve standing. When you are talking to someone, stand well, erect and tall. Don't keep shifting your weight from one foot to the other, or throw it all onto one hip, which pushes your spine out of alignment; but keep it distributed evenly. The way that you stand has a powerful effect on your personality and on your emotional state; on how you approach and respond to others and on how they respond to you.

The Full Breath

Stand in balance with your feet hip width apart, your pelvis centred, your abdomen and buttocks firm. *Exhale* gently, emptying your lungs.

Turn your arms out from your shoulder sockets so that your palms face outwards and your chest opens.

Inhale as you raise your arms to the sides, simultaneously coming up onto the balls of your feet. Bring your palms together above your head with your arms straight.

Then turn your hands so that the backs come together and the palms face the floor.

Exhale controlling the descent of your heels so that they reach the floor at the same time as your arms reach your sides.

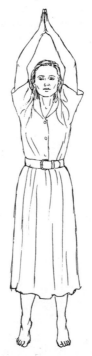

Coordinate the movement with the breath. Be aware of your ribcage extending sideways and upwards against your armpits on each inbreath, and subsiding into its resting position on each outbreath.

Do three to five breaths in all.

The Full Breath can also be practised with the arms raised to the front, which works the intercostal muscles in a different way, and gives a different effect.

Inhale as you raise your straight arms in front until your fingertips point towards the ceiling, simultaneously coming up onto the balls of your feet.

Exhale as you lower your arms to the front and your heels to the floor, coordinating movement with breath.

Make sure that you keep your buttocks squeezed together and your pelvis tucked under so that you avoid over-arching your lower back.

Do three to five breaths in all.

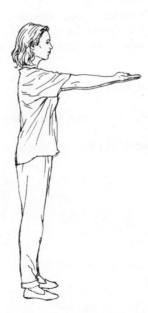

The Sunburst Breath

When we are under a great deal of pressure, we tend to breathe shallowly (and sometimes forget to breathe at all!). At such times, it is helpful to empty the lungs completely with a full, conscious, deliberate exhalation.

The sunburst breath combines a forceful exhalation with an upward and backward stretch, and is a marvellous tension-chaser.

Stand in balance with your feet hip width apart. Squeeze your buttocks together and tuck your pelvis under you.

Inhale and raise your arms in front, keeping them parallel, until your fingertips point towards the ceiling. Palms face forward. Stretch up, and lengthen along your entire body.

Exhale through the mouth with an audible, forceful sigh (say 'AHHH!') as you open your arms wide and stretch backwards. Keep breathing out through the mouth until you feel you can't breathe out any more. Make sure your buttocks stay firmly squeezed: they are essential support for your lower back.

Keep your ears between your arms so you don't contract your neck. Your whole spine should curve smoothly, from your tailbone to the top of your neck. You shouldn't feel any pressure in your lower back.

Inhale and straighten up, stretching fully upwards again.

Exhale and lower your arms to the front.

This is one round. Do three to five in all.

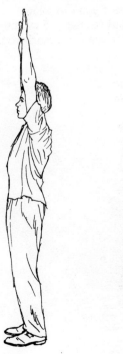
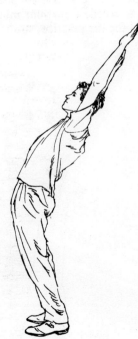

The nine pacifying breaths

This is a lovely sequence, performed with three different movements of the arms: four circular, three triangular, and two parallel, all coordinated with full, deep, slow breaths. It has a calming effect on the nervous system, and will leave you feeling balanced and centred, ready to take control. It's good to practise this before going into any situation that makes you feel anxious – an important meeting or interview, for example – and afterwards, too, to calm you down if you need calming down.

Note: with this, or any other breathing exercise that involves more than a few full breaths, you should stop if you feel dizzy or light-headed.

Stand in balance, and take a few easy, normal breaths to prepare yourself. It helps to close your eyes. See if you can allow everything else to recede from your mind for the two minutes or so you will need for the practice, so that you can absorb yourself in it completely.

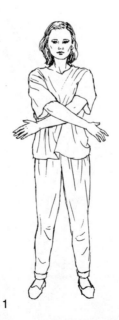

1

First *exhale* gently and take your arms out to the sides a little way, with the backs of your hands facing forward.

Inhale as you cross your arms in front of your body, and lift them (illustration 1). (Imagine you are trying to take a tight pullover off over your head! This will get you to use all the muscles of your trunk – especially your intercostal muscles.)

When your arms are straight up over your head, turn your palms to face the floor.

Exhale as you bring your arms down by your sides and then in front of you (illustration 2). Without stopping the movement or breaking your rhythm, cross them smoothly again in front of your body, and begin the next round.

Take three more breaths in this way: four in all.

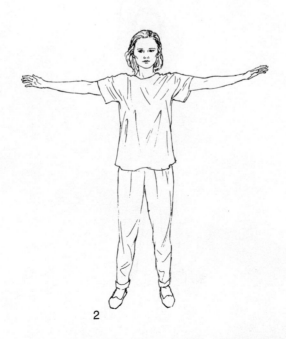

2

Then, with your hands back in their original position a foot or so away from your body, turn the palms to face forward.

Inhale as you raise your arms up and over your head, bringing your palms together (illustration 3). Imagine that you are holding heavy weights in each hand, raising your arms against the resistance of those weights.

Bring the backs of your hands together.

Exhale as you lower your arms to your sides.

Take two more breaths in this way: three in all.

Then turn your hands so that the palms face forwards.

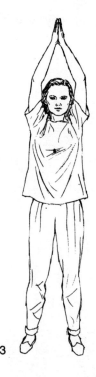

3

Inhale and with the feeling that you are lifting a heavy stone in each hand, raise your arms, keeping them parallel and palms up, until your fingertips point towards the ceiling, palms facing behind you (illustration 4).

Turn your palms to face forward.

Exhale as you lower your arms to the front.

Take one more breath in this way: two in all.

Remain still for a few moments, and observe your breath. You will probably find that you are breathing more slowly, and more deeply, than you were before. When you feel ready to do so, open your eyes.

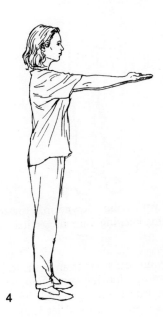

4

Tiptoe Breathing Sequence

Here is another simple sequence, to focus awareness and to encourage the full use of your lung capacity. All the movements are to be coordinated with the breath in a smooth, flowing rhythm.

Stand in balance, with your feet hip width apart and parallel, your pelvis centred and your abdomen and buttocks firm. Take a few normal breaths and feel steady and focused.

Bring the palms of your hands together at the centre of your chest (illustration 1). Gently exhale, emptying your lungs.

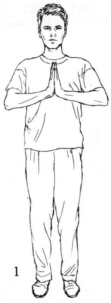

1

Inhale as you direct your palms downwards towards the floor until your arms are straight, keeping your fingertips together (illustration 2).

Exhale as you turn your arms out from your arm sockets so that your palms face forwards, drawing your shoulders back a little (illustration 3). Make this a really graceful, 'opening' movement: feel that your chest is opening up and let your outbreath be long and relaxed.

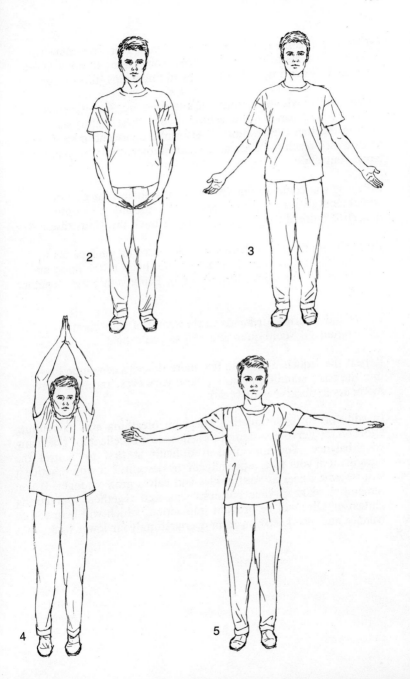

Inhale as you come up onto the balls of your feet, simultaneously raising your arms to the sides to bring your palms together above your head. Stretch up, from toe-tips to finger-tips (illustration 4).

Exhale and slowly lower your heels to the floor, simultaneously returning your hands to the centre of your chest, palms still pressed together (illustration 1). Control the descent of your heels so that they reach the floor at the same moment as your hands reach your chest.

Inhale as you come up onto the balls of your feet once more, straightening your arms upwards, palms still pressed together, fingertips pointed towards the ceiling. Stretch up! (illustration 4)

Bring the backs of your hands together, turning your palms to face out. *Exhale* as you slowly lower your heels to the floor, and your arms to your sides (illustration 5). Bring your palms together in front.

Inhale and return your hands to the centre of your chest (illustration 1). Stand quiet and still as you exhale.

Repeat the sequence three to five more times. Then come back into the basic standing position, close your eyes, and take a few moments to observe your breath.

In addition to its stimulating effect on breathing and its calming effect on the nervous system, this sequence is excellent for practising your balance. You may find it difficult at first to control the movement of your feet, especially on the descent, but with practice it will become easier as your ankles and calves grow stronger. If you remember to keep your buttocks squeezed together, your strong gluteal muscles will be brought into action, which will help you to balance and also keep you from over-arching your lower back.

The Chest Expansion Sequence

This splendid sequence is a real tonic, providing a complete workout for your whole body. It bends the spine backwards and forwards, and stretches the arms and legs. It works all the joints of the fingers, hands and wrists; and digs down deep into the terrible tension pocket between the shoulder blades. Above all, it works the whole of your breathing apparatus, encouraging deeper, fuller respiration and sending a rich supply of fresh oxygen to every cell.

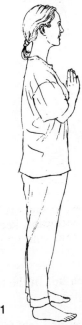

1

Stand in balance with your feet about hip width apart, your pelvis centred and your buttocks and abdomen firm. Bring the palms of your hands together at the centre of your chest (illustration 1).

Exhale and empty your lungs.

Inhale as you push your palms forward and away from you at shoulder level, and then out to the sides in a big, breast-stroke movement. Interlace your fingers behind you at the level of your seat. Lengthen your spine upwards.

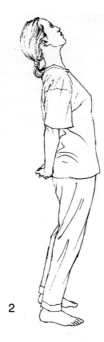

2

Squeeze your buttocks together to support your lower back. *Exhale* as you gently stretch backward, keeping your head in line with your body: don't throw your chin up or tuck it in (illustration 2).

Inhale as you slowly straighten up. In the upright position, lengthen your spine.

Exhale as you bend your knees and fold forwards from your hips, keeping your hands in contact with your lower back (illustration 3).

Lengthen and stretch your spine, and keep your head, neck and spine in line: the crown of your head should face forward and you should be looking at the floor.

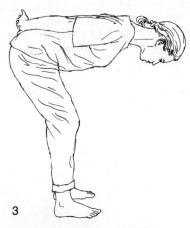

3

Pause when your trunk is parallel to the floor.

Inhale as you squeeze your shoulder blades together and raise your straight arms behind you (illustration 4).

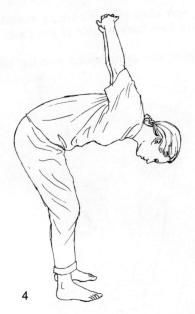

4

Exhale and continue stretching forward from the hips, lengthening your spine (illustration 5). Continue to raise your arms, pressing your hands forward as far as you can without straining. Feel the 'squeeze' between your shoulder blades: it is undoing the tension there.

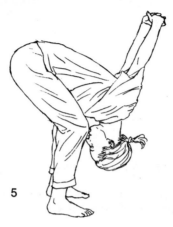

5

CAUTION: the next stage is a very strong stretch which you should omit if you have back trouble of any kind.

Inhale as you slowly start to straighten your legs (illustration 6).

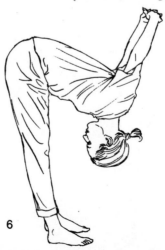

6

Go only as far as you comfortably can: don't feel you have to straighten them fully. Feel the stretch building up from your heels to your buttocks.

Exhale as you hold this position.

Inhale as you bend your knees (illustration 5).

Exhale and, keeping your knees bent, slowly return your trunk to the parallel-with-the-floor position, lowering your arms to rest on your back (illustrations 4 and 3).

Inhale as you come back to the upright position, straightening your legs and keeping your head, neck and spine all in one straight line.

Exhale and squeeze your buttocks together as you gently stretch back (illustration 2).

Inhale as you come upright.

Exhale as you gently release your fingers and sweep your hands round to the front, bringing your palms together.

Inhale as you return your hands to the centre of your chest (illustration 1).

Exhale and stand quietly.

Take a breath or two before repeating the sequence once or twice: more, if you wish to and have the time. Three full rounds should leave you feeling considerably refreshed and revitalized.

Relaxed Standing Forward Bend

This is a lovely, relaxed movement, marvellous for releasing tension in the whole body, especially in the upper back, the shoulders and neck, and the hands and arms.

Stand in balance with your feet hip width apart and parallel, your pelvis centred and your abdomen and buttocks firm. Pull your shoulders down away from your ears and let your arms hang loosely.

Exhale as you tuck in your chin and bend your knees a little, letting the crown of your head move towards the floor (illustration 1). Allow your body to follow your head as you curl down. Keep your chin tucked in so that the back of your neck lengthens. Let your hands and arms dangle loosely (illustration 2).

Curl down as far as you comfortably can, completely relaxing your hands, arms, shoulders and neck. Feel that your entire trunk is heavy and floppy – like a rag doll. Your head should feel heavy too, dangling at the end of your neck like a piece of ripe fruit ready to drop from the branch (illustration 3).

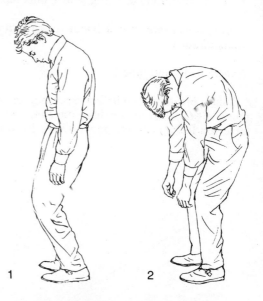

1   2

Inhale as you begin to draw up, keeping your chin tucked in. Use only the muscles of your back to lift your trunk: feel them working, and feel the stretch across the upper and middle areas of your back. Feel that you are drawing something very heavy up out of some very thick mud. Try not to involve your arms and hands: just let them be floppy as they follow your body up.

As you come into the upright position, bend your elbows, bring your loosely curled hands in front of your chest (illustration 4), and gradually start to stretch your arms upwards, above your head. Straighten but don't stiffen your arms, as you direct your fingertips towards the ceiling, palms facing each other.

Stretch up fully, feeling that you are stretching from the soles of your feet to the tips of your fingers – as if you were a rubber band being stretched at both ends, being fully elongated (illustration 5).

Exhale as you curl your hands loosely in front of your face. Bring your elbows close to your chest and tuck in your chin as you begin to curl down once more (illustration 4).

3   4   5

Repeat these movements as many times as you wish, curling down on the outbreath, stretching up on the inbreath. Feel your body growing heavier and floppier and more relaxed with each cycle.

Note: while you are stretching, don't tip your head back: keep looking forwards so that your neck can lengthen, as well as the rest of your spine. And remember to keep your buttocks squeezed together and your pelvis tucked under so that you don't arch your lower back.

You can make this a more dynamic exercise by increasing the speed of the movement and the rate of your breathing. It will then have a more invigorating and stimulating effect. You can also slow it down, taking a few breaths for each movement, and this will make it even more relaxing.

Standing forward bend

In this exercise, you will use a wall to help you stretch and lengthen your spine. It's an excellent ironer-out of knots and kinks in the back, especially in the upper back.

Stand facing a wall, about three feet away from it (the precise distance will depend upon the length of your arms and your upper body). Have your feet parallel and about hip width apart, your pelvis centred and your buttocks and abdomen firm.

Inhale as you raise your arms forward and up until your fingertips point towards the ceiling (illustration 1). Lengthen your spine.

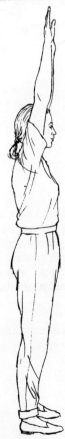

1

Exhale as you bend your knees and fold forwards from your hips, stretching your spine. Don't round your back: keep it long and flat so that you can stretch right from the base of the spine to the back of your neck. Make sure your ears stay between your arms, and stretch your arms, too!

Place your palms against the wall (illustration 2). At this point, adjust your position if necessary. The distance of your feet from the wall should be such that your whole trunk, from your hips to the crown of your head, is parallel to the floor.

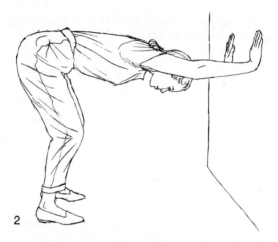

2

Hold this position, keeping your knees bent, and breathe naturally. Push gently against the wall, lengthening your upper back on each inbreath. With each outbreath, allow yourself to release a little bit of the tension you are holding in that area. Feel that your upper back is 'letting go' and releasing down between your shoulders. Your chest and your ribcage should feel open, and your breathing free.

Make sure that your lower back isn't arching. You should feel that you are stretching your whole spine.

CAUTION: omit the next stage if you have back trouble of any kind.

After you have worked in this way for several breaths, slowly begin to straighten your legs (illustration 3) – but only as much as feels comfortable. Keep your pelvis tucked under so that you don't arch your lower back. Feel that you are stretching from the base of your spine to the back of your neck.

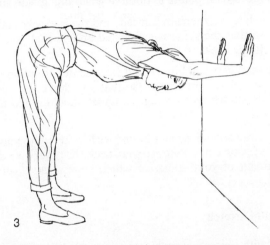

3

After a few breaths, bend your knees and release the presssure of your hands against the wall (illustration 2), but keep your arms straight.

Inhale as you come upright, keeping your ears between your arms. Stretch right up, fingertips pointing towards the ceiling (illustration 1). Keep your buttocks squeezed together and your pelvis tucked under: don't allow your lower back to arch.

Exhale as you lower your arms to the front.

Gently circle your shoulders backwards, and give your arms and hands a shake.

Standing Side Stretches

Stretching sideways creates space between the pelvis and the ribcage, relieving pressure on your abdominal organs and giving them plenty of room to work properly. It opens the ribcage so that you breathe better, and has a marvellous lengthening effect on your entire body, so that you feel better all over.

There are several points to observe when doing side stretches:

- The pelvis must remain centred, and the buttocks and abdomen firm so that the spine is supported and so that you don't arch your lower back.

- Your shoulders and hips should face squarely front and remain in the same plane throughout, so that you don't lose the effect of the side stretch by allowing the upper shoulder and hip to turn forwards.

- Your head should remain in line with your body: you shouldn't tuck in your chin, contract your neck, or otherwise destroy the alignment of your spine (of which your neck is, of course, a part).

Preliminary stretch

Start off with a simple stretching movement which will lengthen you and prepare you for the stronger stretches.

Stand with your feet hip width apart and parallel, your pelvis tucked under, your abdomen and buttocks firm.

Inhale as you raise your arms to the sides and stretch them up above your head until they are parallel with palms facing. *Exhale.*

Inhale as you stretch up along the right side of your body, releasing along the left side. Feel the stretch from the outside of your foot to the tips of your fingers.

Exhale as you release the stretch.

Inhale as you stretch up along the left side, releasing along the right side.

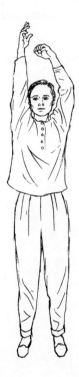

Exhale as you release.

Continue breathing and stretching in this way. Keep your weight evenly distributed on both feet, so that you don't 'kink' on the side you aren't stretching. You should feel that you are elongating both sides of your body.

Finish by stretching up equally on both sides. Hold for a few breaths, and then bringing your arms down by your sides on an outbreath.

Gently circle your shoulders backwards a few times.

Side Stretches

1

Stand in balance with your feet parallel and hip width apart, your pelvis centred and your buttocks and abdomen firm. Draw your shoulders down away from your ears and let your arms hang loosely at your sides.

Exhale as you lengthen upwards, and then stretch over to the right, your whole trunk moving in a smooth curve.

Inhale as you come slowly upright into the central position, keeping your buttocks squeezed together and your abdominal muscles pulled in.

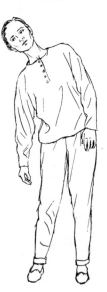

Pause in the central position and lengthen upwards.

Exhale and stretch over to the left.

Inhale and come slowly back to the central position.

Repeat twice more to each side.

Keep your hips stable, and facing forwards: don't allow your left hip to poke out. Go only as far as you can without kinking your left waist: you are *stretching*, not bending.

Don't involve your arms or shoulders: just allow your right hand to slide down your right thigh, and your left hand to slide up your left thigh. Make sure your left shoulder doesn't hunch up: keep a nice, big space between it and your ear.

2
Stand in balance, your feet about eighteen inches apart, your pelvis centred and your buttocks and abdomen firm.

Inhale and raise your arms to the sides, bringing your fingertips together above your head with your elbows bent. Draw your shoulders down away from your ears; direct your elbows back.

Exhale as you curve your upper body slowly over to the right. Visualize a big beach ball or barrel tucked into your right waist: you have to go up and over it.

Keep your left shoulder and elbow well back. At the end of the outbreath, gently pull in on your lower abdominal muscles.

Inhale as you slowly come back up into the central position.

Pause and lengthen up in the central position.

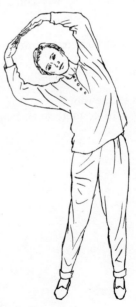

Exhale and slowly stretch over to the left in the same way.

Inhale as you come back up.

Repeat twice more to each side.

3

Stand in balance with your feet hip width apart, your pelvis centred and your abdomen and buttocks firm.

Inhale and raise your arms to the sides and up above your head. Straighten your elbows, interlace your fingers and turn your palms to face the ceiling. Stretch up.

Exhale as you stretch over to the right. Keep your arms straight, your left shoulder well back, and your buttocks and abdomen firm. Again, visualize the barrel or beach ball tucked into your right waist: lengthen up and curve smoothly over it. Pull in on your lower abdominal muscles.

Inhale as you slowly come back to the centre. Pause and stretch up.

Exhale as you stretch over to the left.

Inhale as you come up.

This is one round.
Repeat twice more to each side.

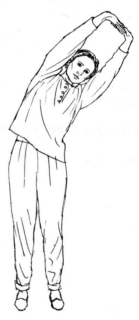

4
This side stretch incorporates a balancing exercise. The starting position and the position of the hands are the same as for the previous exercise.

Inhale and raise your arms to the sides and up above your head. Straighten your elbows, interlace your fingers and turn your palms to face the ceiling. Simultaneously come up onto your toes.

Exhale as you slowly stretch over to the right, remaining up on your toes.

Inhale as you slowly come back to the upright position, remaining up on your toes.

Exhale as you stretch over to the left, remaining up on your toes.

Inhale as you come upright, remaining on your toes.

Repeat once more to each side,
remaining up on your toes.

Exhale as you slowly lower your heels,
simultaneously releasing your
fingers and lowering your arms to
your sides.

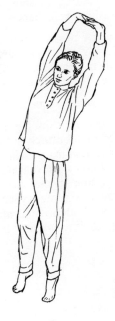

The Buttocks

You will have noticed the recurrent instruction throughout this chapter to squeeze the buttocks together and to hold them firm.

We tend to regard our buttocks as an innocuous mass of flesh, riding along behind us, but they are *muscles*: the largest and strongest in the body; and they need to be used if they are to do their job properly. Their job is to support the pelvis and hold it central; and thus to help support the spine, protecting the lower back in particular from strain and injury. The buttocks also work in conjunction with the abdominal muscles to lift and lengthen the whole upper body.

So be aware of your buttocks when you do the standing exercises, in order to attain optimum length in your spine, and to avoid over-arching it. This is particularly important when you are doing backbending exercises.

You can also find ways of using your buttocks during your activities throughout the day. For example:

- While standing, or doing any activity that requires you to stand, like washing your hands, washing up, house-cleaning, etc.

- If you have to stand in the bus or train on your journey to work, stand with your feet apart, squeeze your buttocks together and hold them firm. This will make it easier for you to keep your balance. Try it without holding onto a railing or strap!

- While walking, squeeze each buttock in turn.

- When you are climbing hills or stairs, or going up the escalator, squeeze each buttock in turn. This will propel you forwards and upwards, making the climb much easier, and avoiding the strain on the lower back that uphill work often places on it.

These simple 'tricks' will help to firm and strengthen your buttock muscles, protect your spine and improve your posture. They will have a cosmetic spin-off too, in firming your buttocks and improving the lines of your body.

Chapter 7
The Beginning, Middle and End of the Working Day

One of the hazards of working life, especially if you have to commute any distance, is the 'tennis ball' syndrome: the feeling that you are constantly being batted to and fro, from home to work and back again. Then self-pity starts to build up because you never have any time for yourself: you always seem to be working or commuting or sleeping.

These are terrible feelings to have, easy to indulge and difficult to control; and they can sap your vital energy and poison your life. The best way I have found to chase them is to get up early to do something I like doing. At different times in my life it has been swimming, running, cycling; and for a number of years now it has been yoga practice. The effort of getting up early is a thousand times repaid: not only by the physical benefits, but by the very fact of having taken that time to do what I want to do, *first* – before heading into the day's commitments and responsibilities.

Even if you are 'no good in the morning', you might just find it possible to get up half an hour earlier, and take that time for yourself. It's your own inviolable space: once you've had it, it can't be taken away from you – and your life will feel less of a treadmill.

Start the moment you wake up: in bed. It's easier to get up and get started if you spend a few minutes stretching even before you get out of bed. Animals do this: you'll always observe cats and dogs stretching themselves after a sleep before getting to their feet and moving around, unless they have been startled or frightened awake. A little stretch in bed will wake up your muscles and get your circulation and breathing going; so that if morning is really a bad time for you, you'll feel a bit less awful. Then, get up and get on with your chosen activity.

The hours you spend travelling to and from your job are very much a part of your working day, possibly the most arduous part. Commuting can be a nightmare, in which you feel you are fighting a losing battle against crowds and dismal travelling conditions; and in which everything conspires to irritate and frustrate you. But you can learn to regard it in a different light: as an opportunity for quiet and reflection.

Unless you really cannot get to work by public transport, it is better to avoid driving. Driving, however used to it you are, and even if you enjoy it, is hard work. You need to concentrate all the time and contend with harassing traffic conditions. Your journeys are bound to be tiring. If you travel by public transport, it is someone else's responsibility to get you to your destination, and you can relax and let them get on with it.

It *is* possible to relax on the train or in the bus: to switch off and turn inward; to replenish your energies instead of squandering them in annoyance at British Rail and outrage at your fellow passengers. You have the choice.

If your train is cancelled, or the bus queue endless, you can practise standing. Remembering the instructions for establishing the basic standing position, employ your waiting time to centre and calm yourself, strengthen your spine and improve your posture. Then the time won't be wasted, and you won't be frustrated.

If, when your transport arrives, you are lucky and get a seat, sit well! Distribute your weight evenly on both buttocks, try not to slump, and avoid crossing your legs, which cuts off your circulation. You can use the time to read, or to think constructively about the day ahead. Or you can simply sit, and breathe.

Here, for example, is a very simple breathing practice, which I think you will find refreshing and relaxing.

Sit well, your lower back firmly up against the back of your seat, your spine straight and long, your feet flat on the floor and hip width apart, your hands relaxed in your lap (or on top of your handbag or briefcase, which will need guarding).

Your hands can be gently clasped, or folded; or you can hold the thumb of one hand lightly in the other hand. Or you can place both hands palms down on the tops of your thighs. Do whichever feels most comfortable for you.

First, just listen to all the sounds around you. Don't try to ignore them or shut them out: be aware of as many sounds as possible, both inside and outside your vehicle.

Then, focus on just one sound, letting all the others recede.

Finally, let all the sounds recede and form a background, from which you yourself are detached.

Begin to focus your awareness on your breath, and watch each inbreath and each outbreath.

When it feels natural to do so, gently close your eyes, first blinking slowly once or twice. Soften your gaze behind your closed eyelids.

Observe the temperature of the breath in your nostrils. Observe the passage of the breath as it moves up and down the nostrils. Observe the texture of the breath.

Make no effort to control or regulate your breath: just let it be, and observe it as it is. After a few minutes you will probably notice that it becomes calmer, slower and shallower.

Allow each outbreath to take as long as it needs. Don't prolong it, but also don't force it or hurry it. Just let it flow out. At the end of each outbreath, leave a little space before the next inbreath. You will breathe in when you need to, so just wait for that to happen. In the little space between, just sit quietly.

As each breath flows out, feel that your facial muscles are softening. Feel that your forehead is widening, that the frown lines are being smoothed away, that your eyelids are growing softer, that your cheeks are growing fuller. Feel that your lips are soft: they should be just lightly closed, and your teeth slightly open. Check your tongue: if you find that it is clamped to the roof of your mouth, release it and let it rest gently behind your lower teeth. Just let it be thick and heavy in your mouth.

Then focus your awareness on your hands, and with each outbreath feel that they are growing heavier and quieter. Be very aware of your hands, and of the sensations of stillness and heaviness in them.

Don't attempt to resist the movement of the train or bus. Just allow your body to give to the movement, and to go with it.

Shortly before you reach your destination (or whenever you've had enough), gradually begin to deepen your breathing. Then stretch your fingers and hands, and move your feet. Open your eyes slowly.

When you get up, do it mindfully, disturbing yourself as little as possible. Don't heave yourself out of your seat and rush headlong to the ticket barrier. Move with awareness, keeping the sensations of relaxation and heightened awareness as you continue on your journey.

You may find this practice so relaxing that you fall asleep, particularly on your homeward journey. Be careful not to ride past your stop – and make sure you have collected all your belongings!

When you have to stand, stand well. Plant your feet firmly on the ground, hip width apart or a little more if there is room, and parallel. Squeeze your buttocks together and tuck your pelvis under. Keep your buttocks firm throughout the journey: they will support you and help to keep you upright. Instead of strap-hanging, which will pull your spine out of alignment (especially if you are short), practise holding your balance without using your hands. As your vehicle moves and sways, allow your body to go with it, shifting your weight through your feet to adjust your balance. Allow your knees to 'give' a little, and keep the backs of them soft. Let your shoulders, neck, jaw and tongue be soft.

Possibly you really do have to drive to work. In that case, you will be able to minimize the stresses and strains of your journey to a considerable degree, mainly by observing the principles of good sitting. Make sure that the base of your spine is right up against the back of your seat, so that your back isn't rounded, or your chest collapsed and your abdomen squashed. Make a point of lengthening upwards, consciously lifting your ribcage and drawing your shoulders back and down. Then you will be able to breathe well, and you'll be giving your internal organs room to function. Make sure that your feet are the right distance from the pedals, and your body the right distance from the steering wheel, so that you don't build unnecessary tension in your legs and arms. Hold the steering wheel lightly: gripping it will create tension in your hands, arms, back, neck and jaw. Try not to clench your teeth or drive with your chin!

When you are stopped at a traffic light, or stuck in traffic, accept that there is nothing you can do to speed things up. Regard that time as time for yourself, an unexpected gift: use it to switch off and let go. Apply the handbrake and shift into neutral; pull your shoulders down, rest your hands in your lap, and take a few deep breaths. Even a few seconds spent like this will relax you a little – and it will be a much more fruitful use of the time than fuming, ranting, clutching the wheel, and revving the engine; which won't get you to work any faster but will ensure that you are a mass of tension and frayed nerves by the time you do get there.

I've assumed up to now that you have to use transport of one sort or another to get to work, but you are lucky if that isn't the case. Walking is one of the best forms of exercise, and if you can walk all or part of the way to and from work, you'll get fresh air (or at least air) as well as movement. Perhaps, even if you do use public transport, you could get on a few stops further down the line, or get off a few stops earlier.

When you walk, try lengthening your normal stride by just one inch. This is a remarkably effective way to maintain and increase your hip mobility. If you walk a lot, try to avoid carrying heavy briefcases, handbags or shopping, which not only unbalance you but also strain your wrists, elbows and shoulders. A rucksack will save those joints, guard your balance, and make for a more enjoyable walk by leaving your arms free to swing. Shoulderbags, incidentally, are not a very good idea. They nearly always force you to lift the shoulder they ride on.

Consider cycling, if the traffic through which you would have to ride is not too horrendous. I used to do it regularly, but stopped after a minor accident; I don't like recommending it, especially now that the roads of most inner cities are deteriorating at such a rate. The prospect of hurtling into one of London's potholes scares me even more than the traffic. But if you are a good cyclist, and you enjoy it, your journeys will give you plenty of excellent exercise.

Your lunchtime gives you an opportunity to get out of the office and stretch yourself. Perhaps there is a nearby park you could walk in, or a swimming pool, or a leisure centre with lunchtime exercise classes – possibly even yoga classes. Doing something of this sort will make a wonderful space in your day, particularly if your work involves always being at others' beck and call. There is the danger, in this situation, that you'll begin to feel put-upon, which will make you unhappy and affect your work and your relations with others. Doing something for yourself, something you like doing, is the best antidote: again, you've chosen to make a space for yourself, and no-one can take it away from you.

More and more firms are becoming aware of the problems of stress in the workplace, and attempting to find ways of helping their employees with these problems. Why not suggest to your personnel department that they make a room available for exercise and relaxation, and even arrange and subsidize classes?

If you can apply even a few of the suggestions in this and the previous chapters, I think you will find that you reach the end of your day in the office with energy to spare for the rest of your life: the vital part that isn't work. You'll know how you want to use those precious hours, so I'll skip now to the *very* end of the day.

A few slow stretching exercises before you go to bed will calm you and help you to relax. I also find it helpful actually to practise conscious relaxation of muscles for the first ten minutes or so in bed, before going to sleep. When I take the time to do this, my muscles really let go, and I sleep better.

If you'd like to try this, first of all lie down carefully on your back, without 'plunking' yourself. Make sure that your whole body is in line. Gently stretch your heels away from you, and stretch your fingers and hands. Draw your shoulders down away from your ears. Rest your hands comfortably on your abdomen or your ribcage, and have your elbows far enough out from your body so that your shoulders can let go. Your upper back should feel wide, and your chest open.

Become aware of your breath, and observe it as it begins to settle and slow down. On each outbreath, let go of a little bit of tension: feel it flowing out of your body with the breath.

Mentally go through your body beginning with your toes, feet and legs; continuing with your fingers, hands and arms; your torso, and finally your face: your forehead, your eyelids, your nose, your cheeks, your lips, your teeth, your tongue and your jaw and throat. With each outgoing breath, let go of tension in that part of the body. If your tongue is clamped to the roof of your mouth, release it and let it rest on the bottom of your mouth, just behind your lower teeth, feeling thick, wide and heavy.

After ten minutes or so, your muscles will have surrendered a great deal of their tension, and will allow you to experience a sounder and more restful night's sleep. (By that time you may well have fallen asleep anyway!)

The time you spend watching television can be used to practise sitting well in your chair (instead of slouching!). Better still, sit cross-legged on the floor to give your hips a passive workout. Place a firm cushion, or some telephone directories, under your buttocks to ease the strain on your lower back and to allow your knees to touch the floor, and work on lengthening your spine.

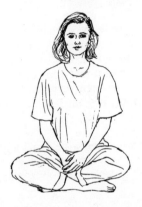

Or you can sit (on your sitting bones) with your legs outstretched in front of you, and your hands resting comfortably in your lap, and stretch your spine. By stretching your heels away from you you can also stretch the backs of your legs. If you find this uncomfortable at first, elevate your buttocks to reduce the strain on your back until the muscles are stronger. They will be if you practise this exercise: it's a great back strengthener.

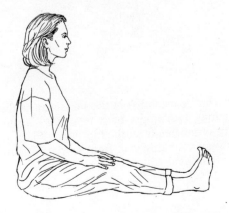

Sitting in this position, you can do all the exercises for the toes, ankles and knees, fingers, wrists and elbows described in Chapter 4. If you find this a strain on your back, you can lean slightly back from your hips, placing your hands on the floor beside your hips or slightly behind them for support while you do your toes, ankles and knees. But make sure that you keep your spine long and upright: don't allow it to collapse.

You can extend this exercise by stretching your upper body forwards, moving it from the hips. Don't be tempted to round your back in an effort to 'go further', but keep your whole spine in a good straight line, and direct your chest forwards rather than downwards. Increase the stretch very gently and very gradually: don't force it. Remember: it's not how far you go, but *how* you go that is important.

You can also sit with your legs wide apart and your heels stretched away. This stretches the adductor muscles of the insides of your thighs, as well as stretching your spine and strengthening your back.

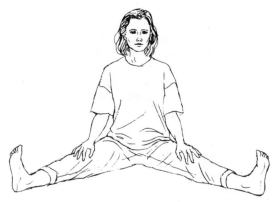

This exercise can be extended in the same way as the previous one, by stretching your upper body forwards – again making sure the movement originates from the hip joints. Place your hands on the floor between your thighs in front of you. Again, increase this stretch gently and gradually.

Finally, here are two exercises to open your hip joints and increase their mobility, which are nice to do in front of the television. These stretch your spine too!

1

Sit on your sitting bones with your legs outstretched in front of you, and lengthen your spine. Bend both your knees up and bring your heels as close as possible to your buttocks. Then allow your knees to drop towards the floor, and bring the soles of your feet together. Take hold of your ankles, one in each hand, and gently press with your elbows on your inner thighs to encourage your knees towards the floor. (Don't press so hard that you strain your knees: if you feel pain or discomfort, go easier.) Sit with your spine upright, and keep lengthening it upwards as you direct your knees towards the floor.

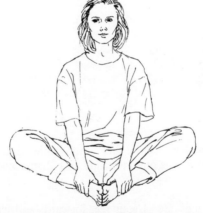

Sit like this for as long as you feel comfortable. Then gently release your ankles and carefully lift your knees, placing your hands under their sides for support. Straighten your legs and circle your ankles.

You can extend this exercise by clasping your hands around your toes, but only if this doesn't cause your back and your chest to collapse. If it does, return to holding your ankles.

When this position feels easy and comfortable, you can extend it further by stretching gently forwards from the hips, as in the previous two exercises.

2

Sit as before with your legs outstretched in front of you, and lengthen your spine. Bend your left knee and bring your heel right into your groin, placing the sole of the foot against the inside of your right thigh. Bend your right knee and fold the leg back, bringing the foot close to your right buttock. Rest your hands comfortably on your knees, lengthen your spine and breathe steadily.

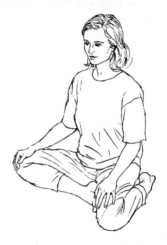

Sit like this for as long as you feel comfortable, and then carefully straighten out your legs one at a time and change over to the other side.

Straighten your legs. Bend your feet forwards and backwards a few times, and circle your ankles.

With these exercises, you can put in a good half hour to an hour's practice while watching your favourite programme – and instead of feeling cramped and lethargic when it's over, you will be beautifully stretched and opened up.

Chapter 8
Using this book throughout your day

Once you have worked with this book for a while and are familiar with the exercises, you will be increasingly able to choose just which ones you need when you need them. You will also become more aware of how you are feeling throughout the day, and will usually know what to do to undo tension and relieve stress.

The purpose of this chapter is twofold: to start you off by suggesting suitable exercises for specific situations, and to help in 'emergencies' – by which I mean the times when you are under so much pressure, and possibly so wound up, that you can't think (or can't stop to think) what to do to help yourself.

The most important thing is to put in a couple of minutes every hour or so, so that tension doesn't get a grip on you. It's like a safety valve that releases a little bit of steam at intervals to prevent an eventual explosion.

On waking
Exercises for the toes and ankles

Chapter 4 page 71-73

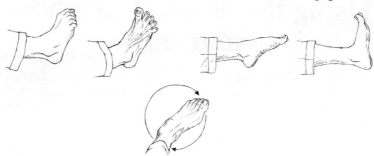

Exercises for the fingers and wrists

Chapter 4 page 63-67

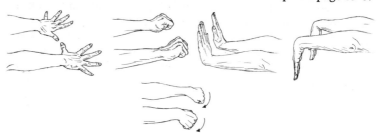

On getting out of bed
Full breath
Chapter 6 page 94

Sunburst breath
Chapter 6 page 96

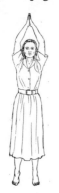

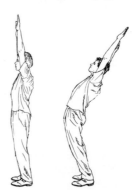

At the bus stop/On the station platform
Standing

Chapter 6 page 90

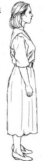

Exercises for the toes and ankles

Chapter 4 page 71-73

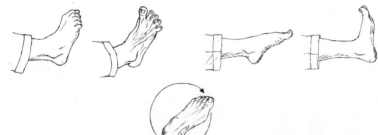

Exercises for the fingers and wrists

Chapter 4 page 63-67

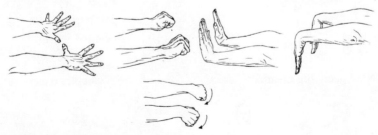

On the bus/train (sitting down)
Breath awareness (2)

Chapter 7 page 124

On the bus/train (standing up)
Standing/balancing

Chapter 6 page 90

136

Before an important meeting or interview, or any situation that provokes anxiety
Breath awareness (1)   Chapter 4 page 80
Full breath   Chapter 6 page 94

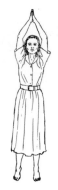

Tiptoe breathing sequence   Chapter 6 page 102

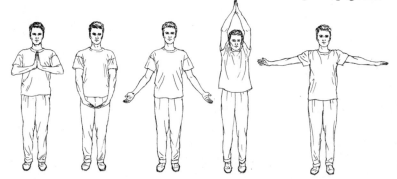

Nine pacifying breaths   Chapter 6 page 98

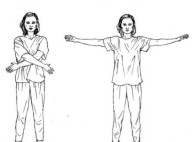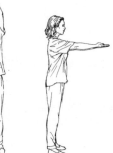

In the meeting
Exercises for the toes and ankles Chapter 4 page 71-73

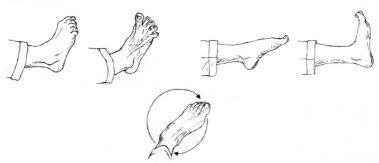

Exercises for the fingers and wrists Chapter 4 page 63-67

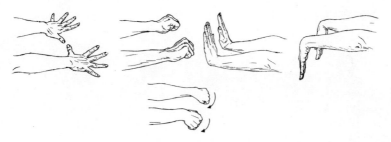

Exercises for the hips Chapter 4 page 76

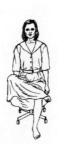

After the meeting
Sunburst breath

Chapter 6 page 96

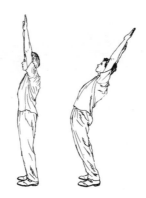

Nine pacifying breaths

Chapter 6 page 98

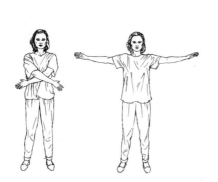
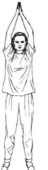

Relaxed standing forward bend

Chapter 6 page 110

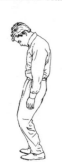
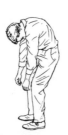

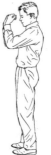
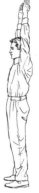

Standing side stretches

Chapter 6 page 116-121

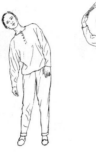 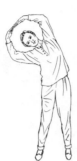 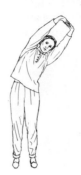

Seated side stretches

Chapter 3 page 56-58

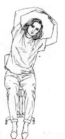 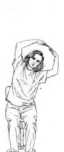 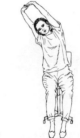

Palming

Chapter 4 page 79

During a prolonged session of writing, typing or word-processing: at frequent intervals

Shoulder circling/	Chapter 2 page 31
Shoulder lifting and squeezing/	Chapter 2 page 32
Shoulder blade squeeze	Chapter 2 page 33

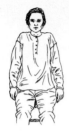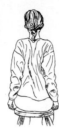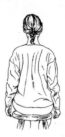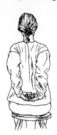

Lowering head forwards/sideways/diagonally   Chapter 2 page 36-38

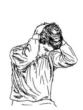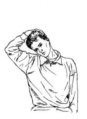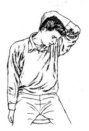

Exercises for the fingers, wrists and elbows   Chapter 4 page 63-69

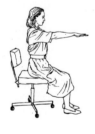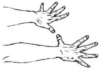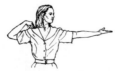

At the end of a long session
Neck and shoulder exercises shown opposite
Stretching spine forwards

Chapter 2 page 31-35
Chapter 3 page 50-51

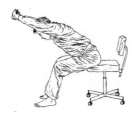 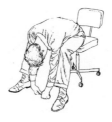

Upper back tension relievers

Chapter 2 page 40-44

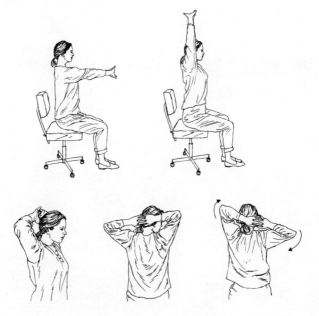

Exercises for the fingers and wrists

Chapter 4 page 63-67

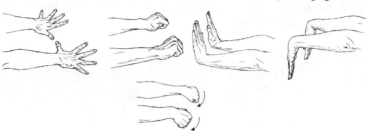

Eye exercises

Chapter 4 page 78-79

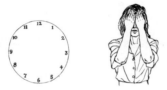

Chest expansion sequence

Chapter 6 page 105

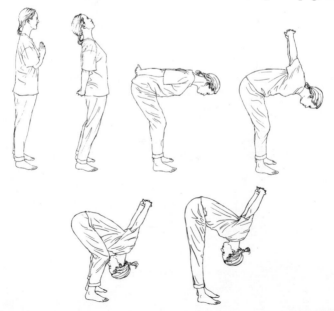

While working fast and under pressure – feeling frantic and breathless
Sunburst breath

Chapter 6 page 96

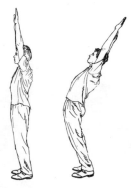

All through the working day
Shoulder circling/
Shoulder lifting and squeezing/
Shoulder blade squeeze

Chapter 2 page 31
Chapter 2 page 32
Chapter 2 page 33

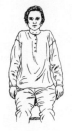 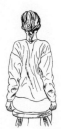 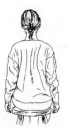 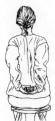

Lowering head forwards/sideways/diagonally   Chapter 2 page 36-38

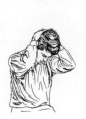 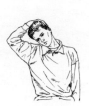 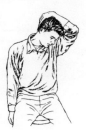

While watching television
Sitting exercises

Chapter 7 page 129-132

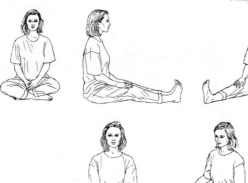
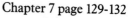

Exercises for the toes and ankles

Chapter 4 page 71-73

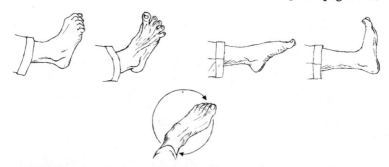

Exercises for the fingers, wrists and elbows

Chapter 4 page 63-67

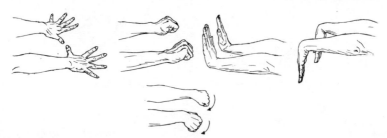

Before bed – to improve sleep
Standing side stretches

Chapter 6 page 116-121

Relaxed standing forward bend

Chapter 6 page 110

Nine pacifying breaths

Chapter 6 page 98

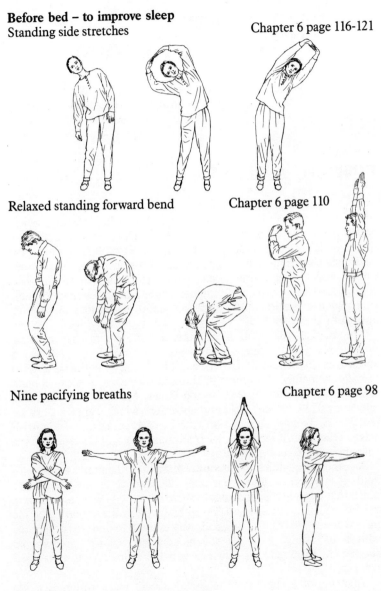

In bed – before/while dropping off
Relaxation

Chapter 7 page 128

Chapter 9
Taking it further

If this book has been your first contact with yoga, and if you have found it helpful, you may want to go further: to attend a class, or practise at home, or – ideally – both. The following notes may be helpful.

FINDING A CLASS

Most local education authorities offer evening yoga classes for adults, and they, or your local library, should be able to provide details of these. You may also be able to find a convenient class at a sports or leisure centre near your home or workplace: quite a few have yoga classes now, as well as the usual aerobics, keep fit, dance, weight and circuit training, etc. Many teachers also run private classes, and some offer individual tuition. Local newspapers, and shops such as health food stores, are good places to look out for notices of these.

The British Wheel of Yoga runs a two-year teacher training programme, and their diploma is recognized by education authorities in Britain and overseas. The Wheel should be able to provide the names of teachers working in your area. You can contact them at 1 Hamilton Place, Boston Road, Sleaford, Lincolnshire: telephone 0529-306851. Other organizations which train teachers are the B.K.S. Iyengar Association, the Friends of Yoga, the Scottish Yoga Teachers Association, the Sivananda Yoga Centre and the International Yoga Fellowship.

A teaching qualification is not a guarantee that the person who holds it is a good teacher (nor does the absence of one necessarily mean that a teacher is inadequate: there are gifted teachers who have not been formally trained). It does, however, indicate that he or she has taken the idea of teaching seriously enough to undergo a rigorous course of study, and has been assessed against professional standards. If you have the choice, it is better to learn from a qualified teacher.

Yoga is not a rigid system, and teachers teach differently. No teacher can be the right teacher for everyone, and the right one for you is one whose approach suits you at your own present level of development. You may need to look around a little. If you start a class and find that you are not enjoying it after participating for a few weeks, then try another: you will find one you are happy with before too long.

The best way to tell whether or not a class is right for you is to observe your own feelings and responses during it and after it. During the class you should enjoy the movements, and feel that you are stretching yourself fully, without straining. Your breathing should feel free, not constrained; and you should feel opened up, not constricted, both physically and mentally. You should feel challenged, but safe. A good teacher will be able to help you to work within your own capacity, so that you do feel all these things. You should never feel that you are being exhorted to push yourself beyond your limits. As my first teacher said: 'Effort, yes; pain, no'.

At the end of the class, you should feel calmer and more relaxed, yet at the same time energized and more alert. You shouldn't feel exhausted. Any mild discomfort you may suffer the next day should be the ache of a muscle that has done some work it isn't used to doing; not the pain of a muscle or ligament that has been overstretched.

PRACTISING AT HOME

To get sustained benefit from yoga, and to progress, you really need to practise regularly. It's the consistency with which you practise, more than the amount of time you spend, that is important.

Don't be too ambitious at first: it is much better to start modestly and build up gradually, than to decide you are going to practise for an hour, and then find you haven't got an hour, and end up doing nothing. Ten or fifteen minutes every day is better than an hour once a week. If you start out with ten or fifteen minutes' practice a day, you will probably find that this extends itself naturally. As your body grows used to the movements and postures, and as your mind becomes attuned, you will look forward to your daily session, enjoy the time you spend at it, and increase that time without effort.

PLACE AND TIME

Try to establish a regular routine. Choose a time and a place that suit you, and practise at the same time and in the same place every day.

The place

This should be clean, dry, warm and preferably quiet. It needn't be large: all you need is sufficient room to stretch yourself fully, whether you are standing up or lying down. It should be a space where you can be on your own, relatively undisturbed. Keep it clear so that it is always ready for you, and make it nice for yourself so that you want to be there and look forward to being there. You might like to have plants, flowers, incense, quiet music.

The time

The time should be one you will be able to stick to. So it needs to fit in comfortably with your other activities, and with your own rhythm and your life style.

If you have the choice, the best time for practice is the early morning. Your body is a little stiffer then, but you are mentally fresher and more alert. The demands of the day have not yet begun to impinge, the mind is clear and quiet, and it is easier to concentrate. The air is fresher, too, before the traffic gets going. (If you have a garden, it is especially nice to practise outdoors on a summer morning.) A morning practice session will leave you feeling good for the rest of the day, with more energy to tackle the problems of work and some left over. For these reasons, the early morning is also a wonderful time for a class, if you can find one.

The early evening may be a more suitable time for you. A practice session when you come home from work will untie all the day's knots (though if you have been working with this book, you shouldn't have too many of those). It will relax and refresh you, and restore your energies for the evening ahead.

Be considerate, though: if you live with someone who expects to be eating his or her evening meal at this time, or who has been waiting all day to talk to you, it may not be a very good idea to start disappearing to your room the moment you walk in the door – at least not before getting assent to your new plan! Your chosen time of practice should not promote disharmony in your family or amongst your friends.

If you choose the early evening, your session has to be fitted in before you eat, because yoga should always be practised with the stomach empty.

The late evening is another possibility, as long as at least two hours have elapsed after eating a light meal, four after a heavy one. A session just before bedtime will calm your mind and nerves, ensuring a deeper and more refreshing night's sleep. But don't include too many movements that will fill you with energy and wake you up, such as strong standing stretches and backward bends. Gentle, relaxed movements, such as seated forward bends, and breathing exercises are best at this time. The nine pacifying breaths calm the mind and nerves in a very short time, and it is helpful to practise them just before you go to bed if you suffer from insomnia. (See Chapter 6.)

If you want to devote more time than you can set aside at any one sitting, you might try dividing your practice up, so that you do ten minutes or so in the morning, another ten when you come home from work, and another just before you go to bed.

Don't forget that you can make use of the time you spend journeying to and from work, and that it may also be possible for you to use part of your lunch time for practice, if there is a suitable place for it. (See Chapter 7 for suggestions on making the most of the beginning and end of the day.)

PLANNING YOUR PRACTICE

After their first few lessons, keen students often ask whether there is a book from which they can practise at home. You will find some suggestions in the reading list on page 151, but if you are working with a teacher, it's much better to practise what you have been taught in the class.

At first, you may find it difficult to remember what you've done in class, but after a little while it will all begin to sink in. Start your home practice with what you can remember, gradually introducing new things as soon as you feel confident about them. Your teacher may be willing to start you off by suggesting a home practice plan of your own.

Your practice should be balanced, and should include a range of movements for the spine (a forward stretch, a backward stretch, a side stretch and a twisting movement). It should also include an inversion of the body (in which the head is lower than the heart) and a balancing exercise.

Start, and finish, your practice with a few minutes of relaxation. The initial relaxation is for quieting down, making a space, establishing breath awareness, and centring yourself before beginning to move your body. The relaxation at the end consolidates the effects of everything you have done in your session.

Make sure you have at hand something warm to put on, as the body temperature drops during relaxation and unless the room you are working in is very warm, you may feel cold.

General points

- When you practise, you should wear comfortable, non-restrictive clothing in which your whole body is free to move. Track suits, or loose trousers and T-shirts, are ideal for both men and women; but if you prefer to wear a leotard the tights should be footless, as you need to work barefoot. Nothing should fit tightly, especially around the waist.

- Put your wholehearted effort into your practice, but never strain. Always work slowly and gently, and with respect for your body; and remember that pain is always a signal to stop.

- Remember that muscular stiffness develops, and habits of tension become ingrained, over a long period of time. They will take time to change, so don't be impatient with yourself.

- Work in a relaxed manner, within your own capacity. You don't have to 'get anywhere'. Yoga is not a competition, even with yourself; and you aren't aiming to achieve, but rather to learn to use your body correctly and to quiet your mind.

- Don't hurry from one movement or posture to the next: take time between them to observe their effects.

- Practise for the sake of the practice, and enjoy it. There should be no expectation of results, and no worries.

- Stretching is the key both to relieving tension and releasing energy. In yoga, you stretch not just your muscles, you stretch your whole self. Yoga works to bring about harmony and balance on all levels: physical, emotional, mental and spiritual.

- If you are in doubt regarding the advisability of your doing a particular movement or posture, ask your teacher. If you do not have a teacher, and aren't sure, leave it out.

- If you have any serious health problems – for example, heart trouble, high blood pressure, or spinal problems – or if you are pregnant, please consult your doctor before commencing yoga. You should also make every effort to find a good teacher and follow his or her advice, rather than practise entirely on your own.

Reading List

Yoga is a practical science. You cannot really learn it from books, but only through practice and experience.

But it is also a subject of tremendous breadth and depth, covering every aspect of human existence, and many good books have been written about it. Books can spark questions in your mind and open up new avenues for exploration and discovery. If your interest in yoga deepens, you may find reading about it a useful adjunct to your practice, as well as enjoyable and enlightening.

This list is a personal selection of some of the books I have found helpful, and can recommend. Not all of them are currently in print, but second hand copies can often be found of those that aren't. Your local library may be willing to order books for you if they don't have them on their shelves.

INTRODUCTORY AND GENERAL BOOKS

The best way to make progress in yoga is to find a teacher and practise what you are taught by the teacher. If this is really not possible for you, and you want to learn from a book, you should realize that many of the practical instruction books on the market are not suitable for beginners. You will be able to identify them by their illustrations. If the pictures show models with their legs wrapped round their ears, or balancing on their forearms with their backs arched and their feet touching the back of their head, you would do better to avoid that book. If you attempt the more advanced yoga postures without adequate preparation and instruction, you will not be able to do them correctly, and you may hurt yourself.

Look for books that describe and illustrate simple movements and postures. Here are a few that are good:

Richard Hittleman
Yoga for Health
Hamlyn Publishing Group, 1971
One of the first popular yoga books to be published in Britain and still one of the best. Clear instructions for a range of basic movements and breathing exercises, with good drawings.

Laura Mitchell and Barbara Dale
Simple Movement: The Why and How of Exercise
John Murray, 1980
Explains the workings of the body clearly and simply, and gives precise, detailed instructions for a series of excellent stretching and strengthening exercises. It concludes with an extremely helpful section on relaxation.

Maxine Tobias and Mary Stewart
Stretch and Relax
Dorling Kindersley, 1985
A sound and attractive book of yoga-based exercises, with excellent colour illustrations and clear, helpful instructions. The authors, both very experienced teachers, show how to adapt the basic stretches to increase or decrease the strength of each.

Sophy Hoare
Yoga
Macdonald Guidelines, 1977
An excellent short introduction to the history and philosophy of yoga plus instructions for a range of classical postures. Beautiful illustrations in colour and black and white, and a helpful glossary.

Tom Macarthur
Yoga and the Bhagavad Gita
The Aquarian Press, 1986
A review of the nature and purpose of yoga, followed by a straightforward modern prose translation of the Bhagavad Gita.

John Stirk
Structural Fitness
Elm Tree Books, 1988

Bob Anderson
Stretching
Pelham Books, 1986

Arthur Balaskas and John Stirk
Soft Exercise
Unwin Hyman, 1989

BOOKS ON HATHA YOGA

There are several different forms of yoga, offering different methods of self-development. Hatha Yoga, the best known in the West, is concerned with the strengthening and refining of the physical body so as to prepare it for the rigours of the further practices, such as meditation. The postures are only a part of Hatha Yoga, and the following books all give a more complete picture.

Hans Ulrich-Rieker (translator)
The Yoga of Light
Unwin Hyman, 1989
A revised edition of this useful translation of the Hatha Yoga Pradipika, the classical manual of Hatha Yoga.

Theos Bernard
Hatha Yoga
Rider, 1982
One of the best books available: Theos Bernard's record of his own experience, working with a teacher in India, of the traditional Hatha Yoga practices. Splendid photographs of the author performing the classical postures.

Swami Satyananda Saraswati
Asana, Pranayama, Mudra, Bandha
Bihar School of Yoga, Monghyr, India, 1983
A manual of the practices of Hatha Yoga. It sets out clearly and in detail the precautions to be observed when doing postures, as well as their possible benefits.

B.K.S. Iyengar
Light on Yoga
Unwin Hyman, 1971

Ian Rawlinson
Yoga for the West
Unwin Hyman, 1988

André Van Lysebeth
Yoga Self-Taught
Unwin Hyman, 1978

THE CLASSICAL TEXTS OF YOGA

The Bhagavad Gita
This is *the* book about yoga, and one of the great books of all time.
Written in Sanskrit around 500 BC, the Gita is a part of the vast
Hindu epic, The Mahabharata. Its message and its wisdom are as
relevant to us today in the West as they were 2,500 years ago in India.
The Gita is available in a large number of translations. The version
by Juan Mascaró (Penguin, 1970) is poetic and readable and has an
illuminating introduction. A new edition of the excellent translation
by S. Radhakrishnan, which was out of print for many years, has
recently been published by Unwin Hyman (Mandala, 1989).

The Upanishads
The Upanishads, the oldest of the classical texts, contain the great
spiritual truths of yoga. They were transmitted orally from teacher
to pupil over many centuries, and written down, in Sanskrit,
between 800 and 400 BC. There are 108 Upanishads. Of the many
editions available, the Penguin, by Juan Mascaró, offers seven of the
major shorter ones and extracts from six of the longer ones, and is
the easiest to find. It is similar in tone and flavour to his rendering of
the Bhagavad Gita, with an equally stimulating introduction. A clear
and accessible translation by Alistair Shearer and Peter Russell, in a
large format edition with beautiful photographs by Richard Lannoy,
is published by Unwin Hyman (Mandala, 1989).

The Yoga Sutra of Patanjali
Written in Sanskrit between 200 BC and 200 AD, this succinct little
book was the first full, systematic exposition of the theory,
psychology and practice of yoga; and it is still regarded as definitive.
Among the many available translations the one by Swami
Prabhavananda and Christopher Isherwood, entitled *How to Know
God*, (Vedanta Publishing, U.S., 1982) is clear and readable and has
a good explanatory commentary. *The Textbook of Yoga Psychology* by
Rammurti Mishra (Julian Press, 1987) is another excellent
translation with a more detailed commentary. *Effortless Being*, a
straightforward modern version by Alistair Shearer with lovely
photographs by Richard Lannoy, is published by Unwin Hyman
(Mandala, 1989).

BOOKS ON MEDITATION

Meditation is not something one does, but something that happens, or that may happen, when one has prepared for it. It cannot really be taught (although you need a qualified teacher to guide you) and no book, however good, can give more than the barest glimpse of it.

There are hundreds of books on meditation, of varying quality and usefulness. Many are less than helpful. The best ones are by experienced practitioners who speak from their own experience.

The following books are sound and interesting, and approach the topic from different points of view.

Michael Eastcott
The Silent Path
Rider & Company, 1989

William Johnston
Silent Music
Fontana, 1976

Ram Dass
Journey of Awakening
Bantam Books, U.S., 1978

Chogyam Trungpa
Meditation in Action
Shambala/Element Books, 1980

Monks of the Ramakrishna Order
Meditation
Ramakrishna Vedanta Centre, 1984

STRESS AND RELAXATION

Herbert Benson
The Relaxation Response
Fontana, 1984

Laura Mitchell
Simple Relaxation
John Murray, 1987